The Definitive Dash Diet Recipes Collection

Super Easy and Affordable Meals to Get in Shape and Enjoy your Diet

Maya Wilson

Table of contents

Sweet Corn Soup

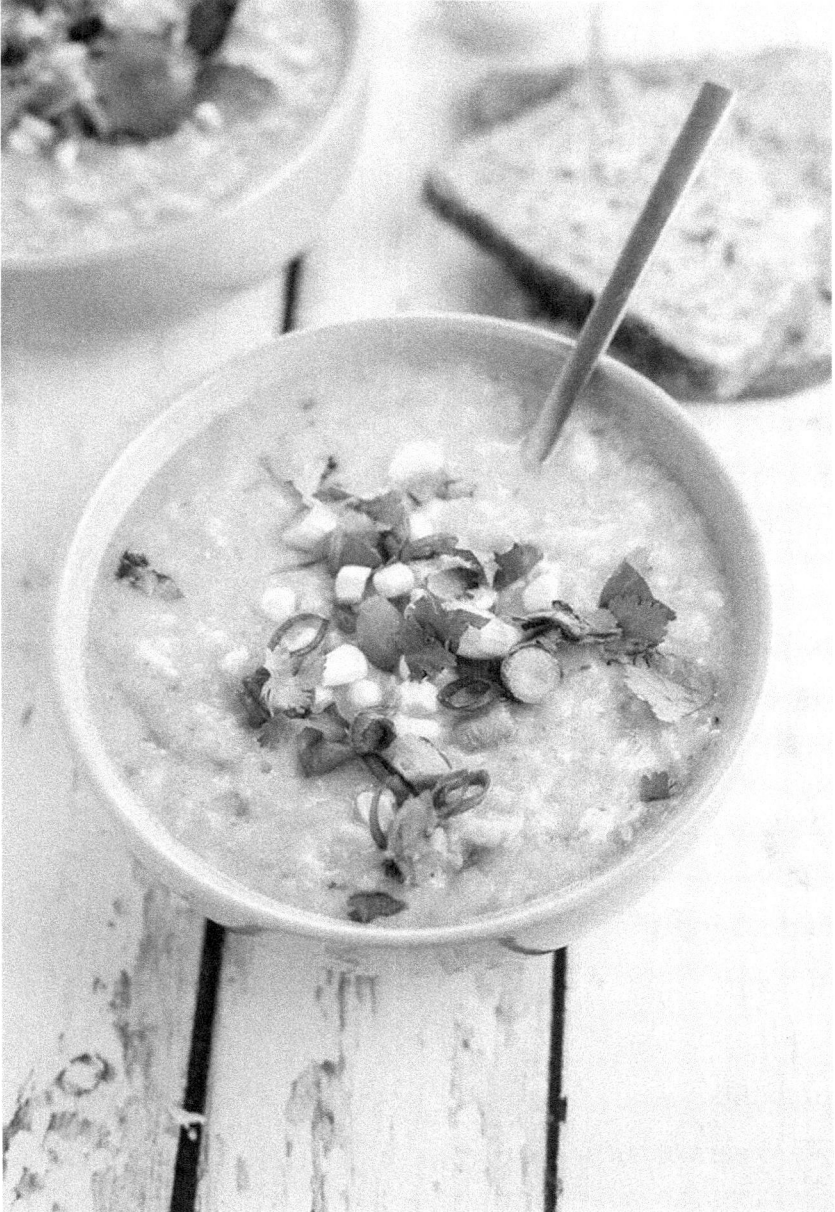

Nutritional Facts

servings per container 4

Prep Total 10 min

Serving Size 2/3 cup (50g)

Amount per serving 120

Calories

% Daily Value

Total Fat 2g 5%

Saturated Fat 0g 8%

Trans Fat 2g 1.20%

Cholesterol 2%

Sodium 16mg 7%

Total Carbohydrate 7g 10%

Dietary Fiber 4g 10%

Total Sugar 12g -

Protein 3g

Vitamin C 2mcg 10%

Calcium 260mg 20%

Iron 20mg 25%

Potassium 235mg 8%

Ingredients

- 6 ears of corn

- 1 tablespoon of corn oil

- 1 small onion

- 1/2 cup grated celery root

- 7 cups water or vegetable stock

- Add salt to taste

Instructions:

1. Shuck the corn & slice off the kernels

2. In a large soup pot put in the oil, onion, celery root, and one cup of water

3. Let that mixture stew under low heat until the onion is soft

4. Include the corn, salt & remaining water and bring it to a boil

5. Cool briefly & then puree in a blender, then wait for it to cool before putting it through a food mill.

6. Reheat & add salt with pepper to taste nice.

Mexican Avocado Salad

Nutritional Facts

servings per container 6

Prep Total 10 min

Serving Size 2/3 cup (70g)

Amount per serving 120

Calories

% Daily Value

Total Fat 8g 10%

Saturated Fat 1g 8%

Trans Fat 0g 21

Cholesterol 22%

Sodium 16mg 7%

Total Carbohydrate 7g 13%

Dietary Fiber 4g 14%

Total Sugar 1g -

Protein 2g

Vitamin C 1mcg 1%

Calcium 260mg 20%

Iron 2mg 25%

Potassium 235mg 6%

Ingredients

- 24 cherry tomatoes, quartered

- 2 tablespoon extra-virgin olive oil

- 4 teaspoons red wine vinegar

- 2 teaspoon salt

- ¼ teaspoon freshly ground black pepper

- Gently chopped ½ medium yellow or white onion

- 1 jalapeño, seeded & finely chopped

- 2 tablespoons chopped fresh cilantro

- ¼ medium head iceberg lettuce, cut into ½-inch ribbons Chopped

- 2 ripe Hass avocados, seeded, peeled

Instructions:

1.   Add tomatoes, oil, vinegar, salt, & pepper in a neat medium bowl. Add onion, jalapeño & cilantro; toss well

2. Put lettuce on a platter & top with avocado

3. Spoon tomato mixture on top and serve.

Crazy Delicious Raw Pad Thai

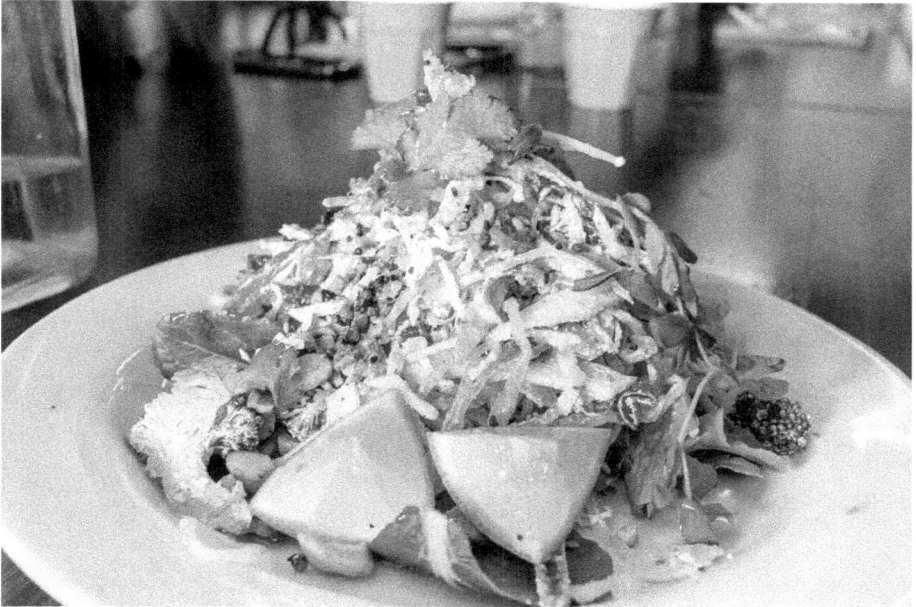

ù

Nutritional Facts

servings per container   3

Prep Total   10 min

Serving Size 2/3 cup (77g)

Amount per serving 210

Calories

     % Daily Value

Total Fat 3g 10%

Saturated Fat 2g   8%

Trans Fat 7g -

Cholesterol   0%

Sodium 120mg   7%

Total Carbohydrate 77g   10%

Dietary Fiber 4g   14%

Total Sugar 12g   -

Protein 3g

Vitamin C 1mcg   20%

Calcium 260mg   20%

Iron 2mg   41%

Potassium 235mg   1%

Ingredients

- 2 large zucchini

- Thinly sliced ¼ red cabbage

- Chopped ¼ cup fresh mint leaves

- Sliced 1 spring onion

- peeled and sliced ½ avocado

- 10 raw almonds

- 4 tablespoonful sesame seeds Dressing

- ¼ cup peanut butter

- 2 tablespoonful tahini

- 2 lemon, juiced

- 2 tablespoonful tamari / salt-reduced soy sauce and add ½ chopped green chili

Instructions:

1. Collect dressing ingredients in a container

2. Pop the top on and shake truly well to join. I like mine pleasant and smooth however you can include a dash of sifted water on the off chance that it looks excessively thick.

3. Using a mandoline or vegetable peeler, expel one external portion of skin from every zucchini and dispose of.

4. Combine zucchini strips, cabbage & dressing in a vast blending bowl and blend well

5. Divide zucchini blend between two plates or bowls

6. Top with residual fixings and appreciate!

Kale And Wild Rice Stir Fly

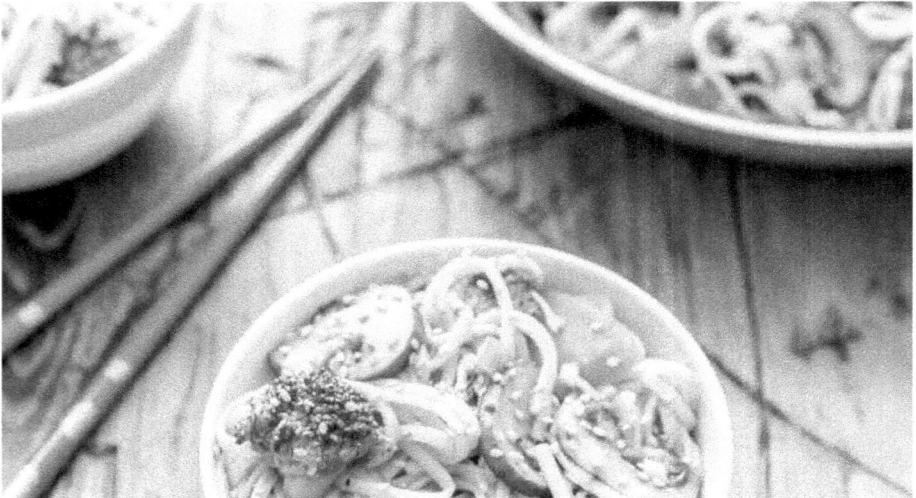

Nutritional Facts

servings per container   3

Prep Total   10 min

Serving Size 2/3 cup (80g)

Amount per serving 220

Calories

% Daily Value

Total Fat 5g   22%

Saturated Fat 1g   8%

Trans Fat 0g -

Cholesterol   0%

Sodium 200mg   7%

Total Carbohydrate 12g   2%

Dietary Fiber 1g   14%

Total Sugar 12g   -

Protein 3g

Vitamin C 2mcg   10%

Calcium 20mg   1%

Iron 2mg   2%

Potassium 235mg   6%

Ingredients

- 1 tablespoonful extra virgin olive oil

- Diced ¼ onion

- 3 carrots, cut into ½ inch slices

- 2 cups assorted mushrooms

- 2 bunch kale, chopped into bite-sized pieces

- 2 tablespoonful lemon juice

- 2 tablespoonful chili flakes, more if desired

- 1 tablespoon Braggs Liquid Aminos

- 2 cup wild rice, cooked

Instructions:

1.	In a large sauté pan, heat oil over on heater. Include onion & cook until translucent, for 35 to 10 minutes.

2.	Include carrots & sauté for another 2 minutes. Include mushrooms & cook for 4 minutes. Include kale, lemon juice, chili flakes & Braggs. Cook until kale is slightly wilted.

3.	Serve over wild rice and enjoy your Lunch!

Creamy Avocado Pasta

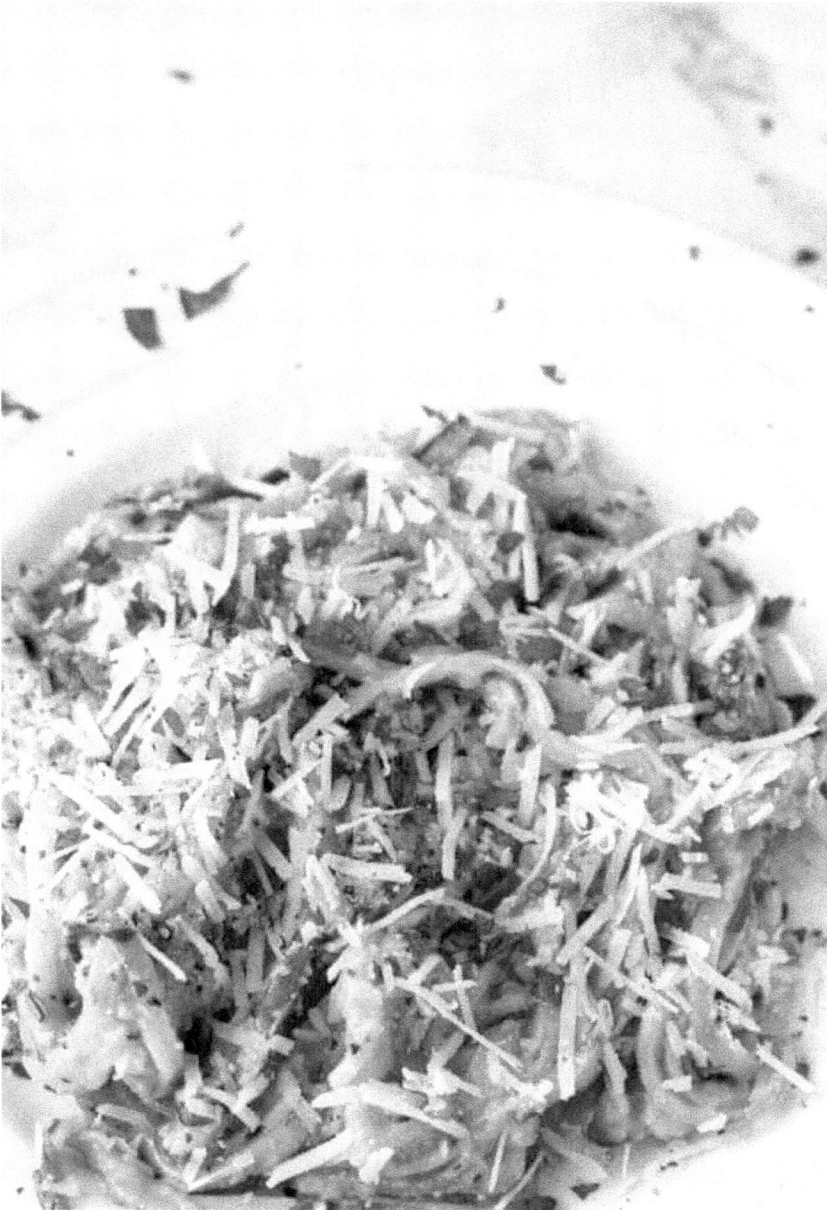

Nutritional Facts

servings per container 7

Prep Total 10 min

Serving Size 2/3 cup (25g)

Amount per serving 19

Calories

% Daily Value

Total Fat 8g 300%

Saturated Fat 1g 40%

Trans Fat 0g 20%

Cholesterol 6%

Sodium 210mg 3%

Total Carbohydrate 22g 400%

Dietary Fiber 4g 1%

Total Sugar 12g 02.20%

Protein 3g

Vitamin C 2mcg 20%

Calcium 10mg 6%

Iron 4mg 7%

Potassium 25mg 6%

Ingredients

- 340 g / 12 oz spaghetti

- 2 ripe avocados, halved, seeded & neatly peeled 1/2 cup fresh basil leaves

- 3 cloves garlic

- 1/3 cup olive oil

- 2-3 teaspoon freshly squeezed lemon juice

- Add sea salt & black pepper, to taste

- 1.5 cups cherry tomatoes, halved

Instructions:

1.   In a large pot of boiling salted water, cook pasta according to the package. When al dente, drain and set aside.

2. To make the avocado sauce, combine avocados, basil, garlic, oil, and lemon juice in food processor. Blend on high until smooth. Season with salt and pepper to taste.

3. In a large bowl, combine pasta, avocado sauce, and cherry tomatoes until evenly coated.

4. To serve, top with additional cherry tomatoes, fresh basil, or lemon zest.

5. Best when fresh. Avocado will oxidize over time so store leftovers in a covered container in refrigerator up to one day.

Black Bean Vegan Wraps

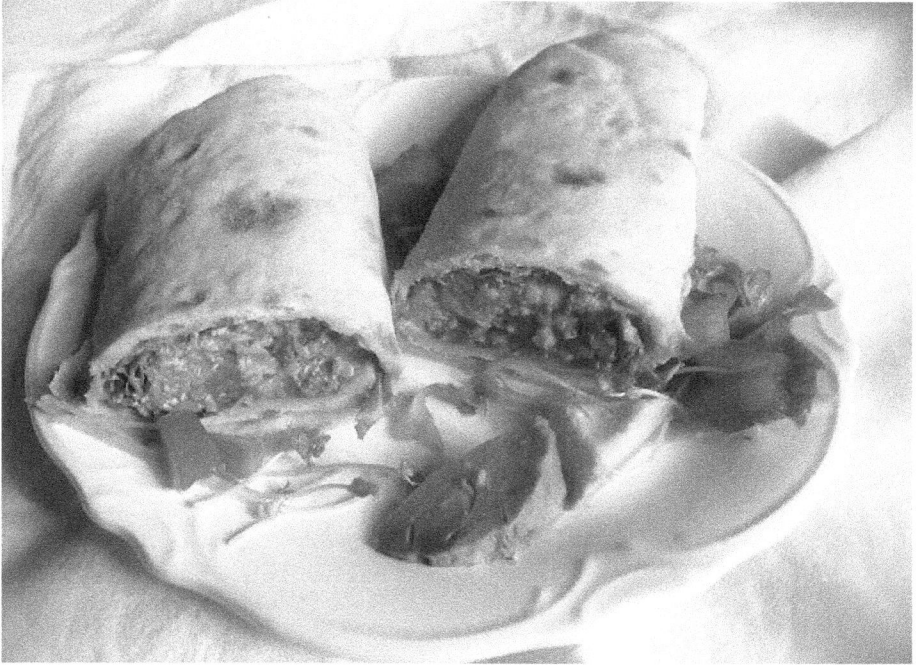

Nutritional Facts

servings per container   5

Prep Total   10 min

Serving Size 2/3 cup (27g)

Amount per serving 200

Calories

     % Daily Value

Total Fat 8g   1%

Saturated Fat 1g   2%

Trans Fat 0g 2%

Cholesterol   2%

Sodium 240mg   7%

Total Carbohydrate 12g   2%

Dietary Fiber 4g   14%

Total Sugar 12g   01.21%

Protein 3g

Vitamin C 2mcg   2%

Calcium 20mg   1%

Iron 7mg   2%

Potassium 25mg   6%

Ingredients

- 1 1/2 half cup of beans (sprouted & cooked)

- 2 carrot

- 1 or 2 tomatoes

- 2 avocado

- 1 cob of corn

- 1 Kale

- 2 or 3 sticks of celery

- 2 persimmons

- 1 Coriander

Dressing:

- 1 hachiyapersimmon (or half a mango)

- Juice of 1 lemon

- 2 to 3 tablespoons original olive oil

- 1/4 clean cup water

- 1 or 2 teaspoons grated fresh ginger

- 1/2 teaspoon of salt

Instructions:

1.   Sprout & cook the black beans

2.   Chop all the ingredients & mix them in a neat bowl with the black beans

3.   Mix all the ingredients for the dressing & pour into the salad

4.   Serve a spoonful in a clean lettuce leaf that you can easily roll into a wrap. Most people do use iceberg or romaine lettuce.

Fascinating Spinach and Beef Meatballs

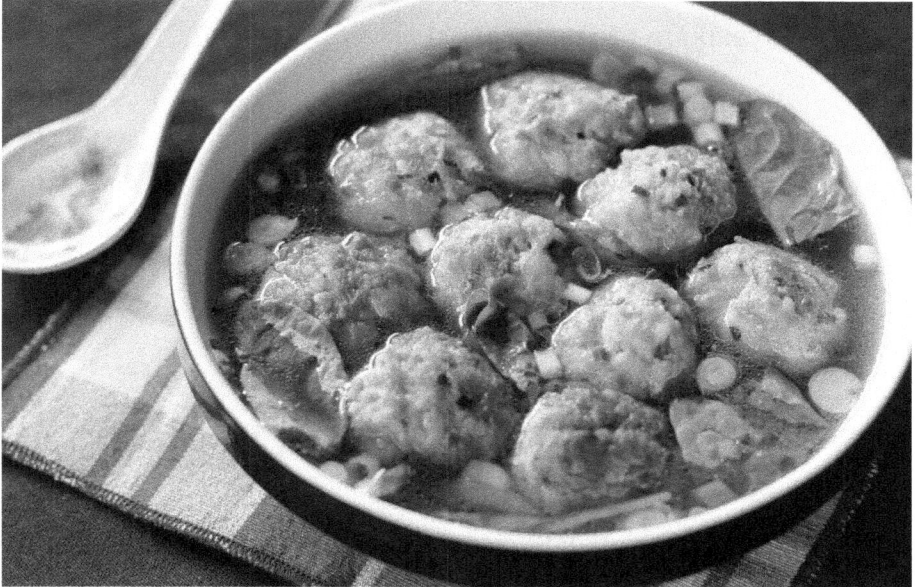

Serving: 4

Prep Time: 10 minutes

Cook Time: 20

Ingredients:

- ½ cup onion

- 4 garlic cloves

- 1 whole egg

- ¼ teaspoon oregano

- Pepper as needed

- 1 pound lean ground beef

- 10 ounces spinach

How To:

1.   Preheat your oven to 375 degrees F.

2.   Take a bowl and blend within the remainder of the ingredients, and using your hands, roll into meatballs.

3.   Transfer to a sheet tray and bake for 20 minutes.

4.   Enjoy!

Nutrition (Per Serving)

Calorie: 200

Fat: 8g

Carbohydrates: 5g

Protein: 29g

Juicy and Peppery Tenderloin

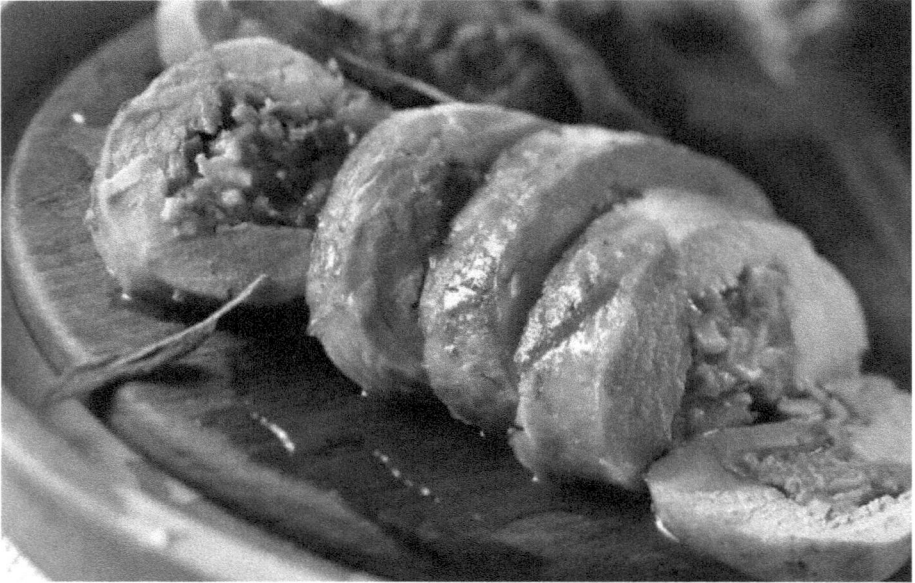

Serving: 4

Prep Time: 10 minutes

Cook Time: 20

Ingredients:

- 2 teaspoons sage, chopped

- Sunflower seeds and pepper

- 2 1/2 pounds beef tenderloin

- 2 teaspoons thyme, chopped

- 2 garlic cloves, sliced

- 2 teaspoons rosemary, chopped

- 4 teaspoons olive oil

How To:

1.   Preheat your oven to 425 degrees F.

2.   Take alittle knife and cut incisions within the tenderloin; insert one slice of garlic into the incision.

3.   Rub meat with oil.

4.   Take a bowl and add sunflower seeds, sage, thyme, rosemary, pepper and blend well.

5.   Rub the spice mix over tenderloin.

6.   Put rubbed tenderloin into the roasting pan and bake for 10 minutes.

7.   Lower temperature to 350 degrees F and cook for 20 minutes more until an indoor thermometer reads 145 degrees F.

8.   Transfer tenderloin to a chopping board and let sit for 15 minutes; slice through 20 pieces and enjoy!

Nutrition (Per Serving)

Calorie: 183

Fat: 9g

Carbohydrates: 1g

Protein: 24g

Healthy Avocado Beef Patties

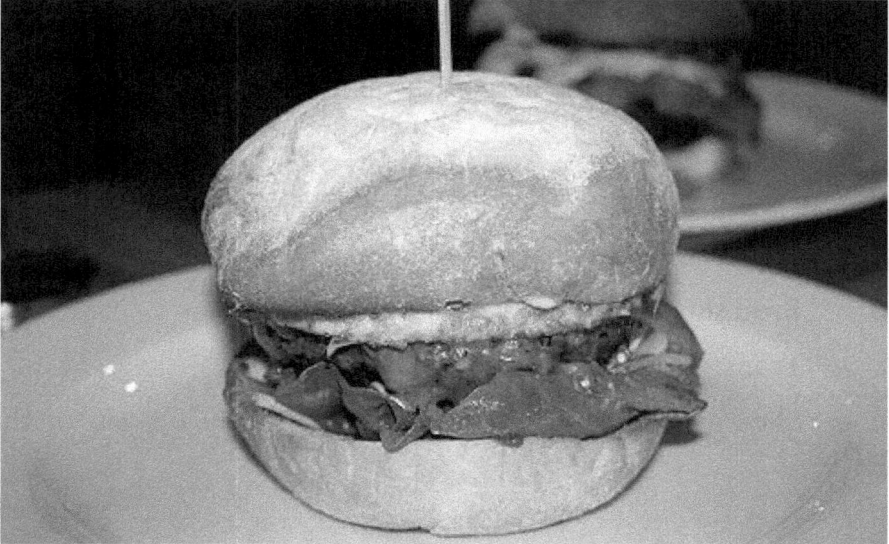

Serving: 2

Prep Time: 15 minutes

Cook Time: 10 minutes

Ingredients:

- 1 pound 85% lean ground beef

- 1 small avocado, pitted and peeled

- Fresh ground black pepper as needed

How To:

1.   Pre-heat and prepare your broiler to high.

2.   Divide beef into two equal-sized patties.

3.   Season the patties with pepper accordingly.

4.   Broil the patties for five minutes per side.

5.   Transfer the patties to a platter.

6.   Slice avocado into strips and place them on top of the patties.

7.   Serve and enjoy!

Nutrition (Per Serving)

Calories: 568

Fat: 43g

Net Carbohydrates: 9g

Protein: 38g

Ravaging Beef Pot Roast

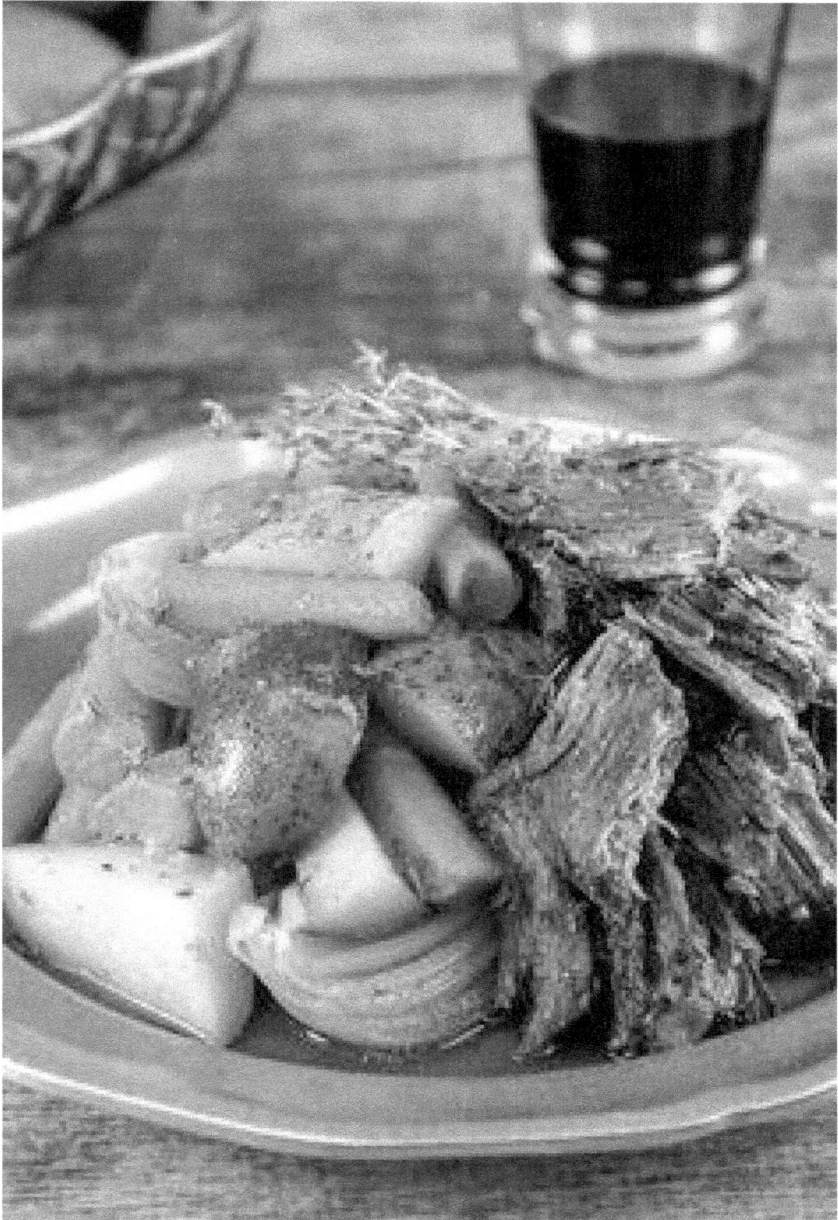

Serving: 4

Prep Time: 10 minutes

Cook Time: 75 minutes

Ingredients:

- 3 ½ pounds beef roast

- 4 ounces mushrooms, sliced

- 12 ounces beef stock

- 1-ounce onion soup mix

- ½ cup Italian dressing, low sodium, and low fat

How To:

1. Take a bowl and add the stock, onion soup mix and Italian dressing

2. Stir.

3. Put roast beef in pan.

4. Add mushrooms, stock mix to the pan and canopy with foil.

5. Preheat your oven to 300 degrees F.

6. Bake for 1 hour and quarter-hour .

7. Let the roast cool.

8. Slice and serve.

9. Enjoy with the gravy on top!

Nutrition (Per Serving)

Calories: 700

Fat: 56g

Carbohydrates: 10g

Protein: 70g

Lovely Faux Mac and Cheese

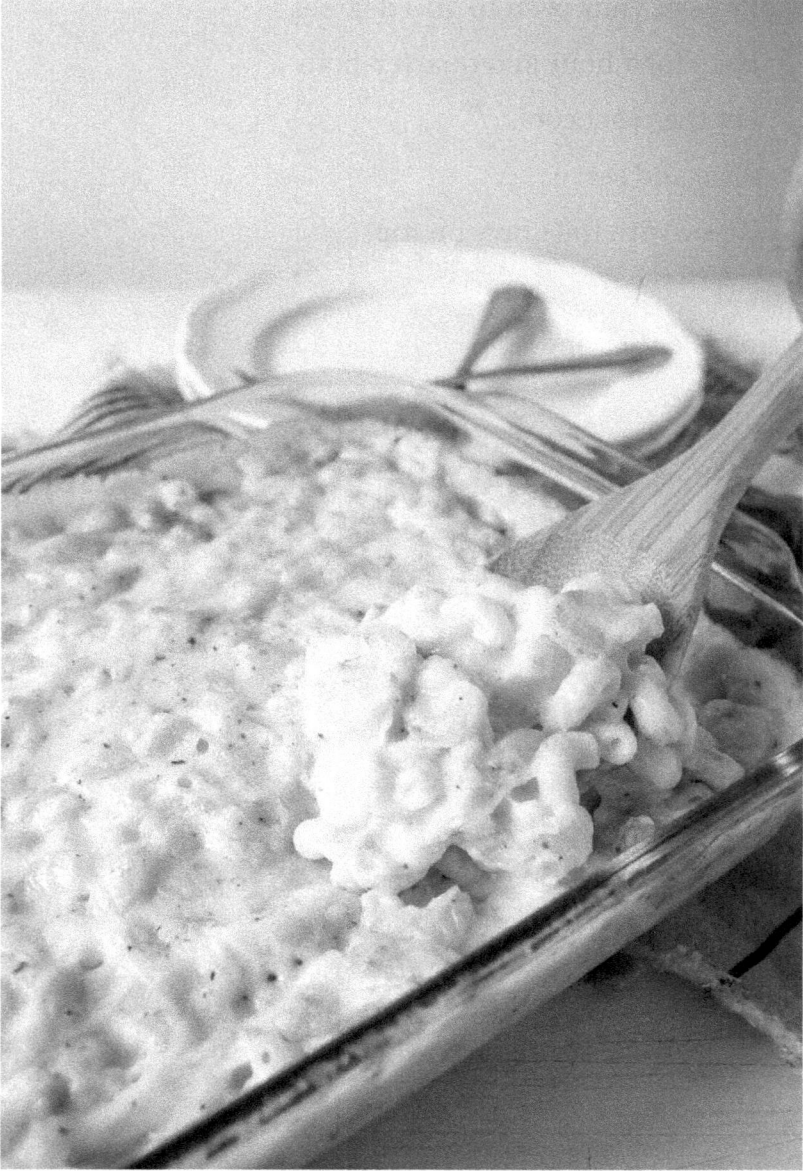

Serving: 4

Prep Time: 15 minutes

Cook Time: 45 minutes

Ingredients:

- 5 cups cauliflower florets

- Sunflower seeds and pepper to taste

- 1 cup coconut almond milk

- ½ cup vegetable broth

- 2 tablespoons coconut flour, sifted

- 1 organic egg, beaten

- 1 cup cashew cheese

How To:

1.   Preheat your oven to 350 degrees F.

2. Season florets with sunflower seeds and steam until firm.

3. Place florets during a greased ovenproof dish.

4. Heat coconut almond milk over medium heat during a skillet, confirm to season the oil with sunflower seeds and pepper.

5. Stir in broth and add coconut flour to the combination , stir.

6. Cook until the sauce begins to bubble.

7. Remove heat and add beaten egg.

8. Pour the thick sauce over the cauliflower and blend in cheese.

9. Bake for 30-45 minutes.

10. Serve and enjoy!

Nutrition (Per Serving)

Calories: 229

Fat: 14g

Carbohydrates: 9g

Protein: 15g

Epic Mango Chicken

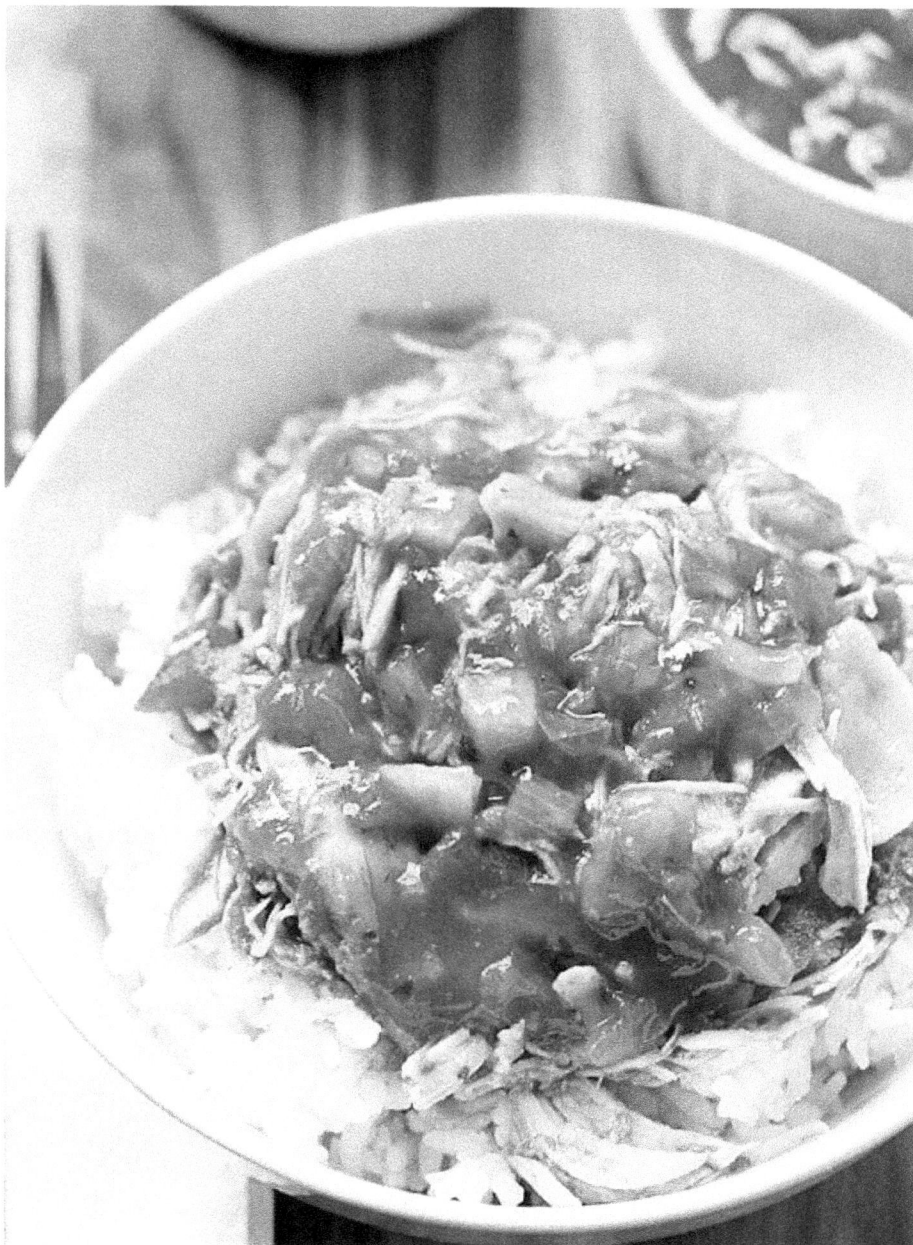

Serving: 4

Prep Time: 25 minutes

Cook Time: 10 minutes

Ingredients:

- 2 medium mangoes, peeled and sliced

- 10-ounce coconut almond milk

- 4 teaspoons vegetable oil

- 4 teaspoons spicy curry paste

- 14-ounce chicken breast halves, skinless and boneless, cut in cubes

- 4 medium shallots

- 1 large English cucumber, sliced and seeded

How To:

1.   Slice half the mangoes and add the halves to a bowl.

2. Add mangoes and coconut almond milk to a blender and blend until you've got a smooth puree.

3. Keep the mixture on the side.

4. Take a large-sized pot and place it over medium heat, add oil and permit the oil to heat up.

5. Add curry paste and cook for 1 minute until you've got a pleasant fragrance, add shallots and chicken to the pot and cook for five minutes.

6. Pour mango puree in to the combination and permit it to heat up.

7. Serve the cooked chicken with mango puree and cucumbers.

8. Enjoy!

Nutrition (Per Serving)

Calories: 398

Fat: 20g

Carbohydrates: 32g

Protein: 26g

Chicken and Cabbage Platter

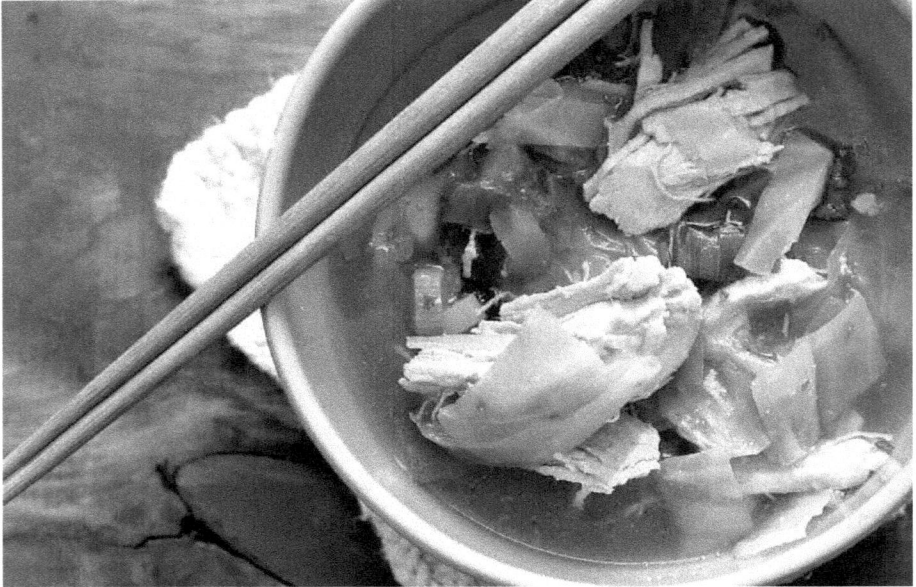

Serving: 2

Prep Time: 9 minutes

Cook Time: 14 minutes

Ingredients:

- ½ cup sliced onion

- 1 tablespoon sesame garlic-flavored oil 2cups shredded Bok-Choy 1/2 cups fresh bean sprouts

- 1 1/2 stalks celery, chopped

- 1 ½ teaspoons minced garlic

- 1/2 teaspoon stevia

- 1/2 cup chicken broth

- 1 tablespoon coconut aminos

- 1/2 tablespoon freshly minced ginger

- 1/2 teaspoon arrowroot

- 2 boneless chicken breasts, cooked and sliced thinly

How To:

1. Shred the cabbage with a knife.

2. Slice onion and increase your platter alongside the rotisserie chicken.

3. Add a dollop of mayonnaise on top and drizzle vegetable oil over the cabbage.

4.   Season with sunflower seeds and pepper consistent with your taste.

5.   Enjoy!

Nutrition (Per Serving)

Calories: 368

Fat: 18g

Net Carbohydrates: 8g

Protein: 42g

Fiber: 3g

Carbohydrates: 11g

Hearty Chicken Liver Stew

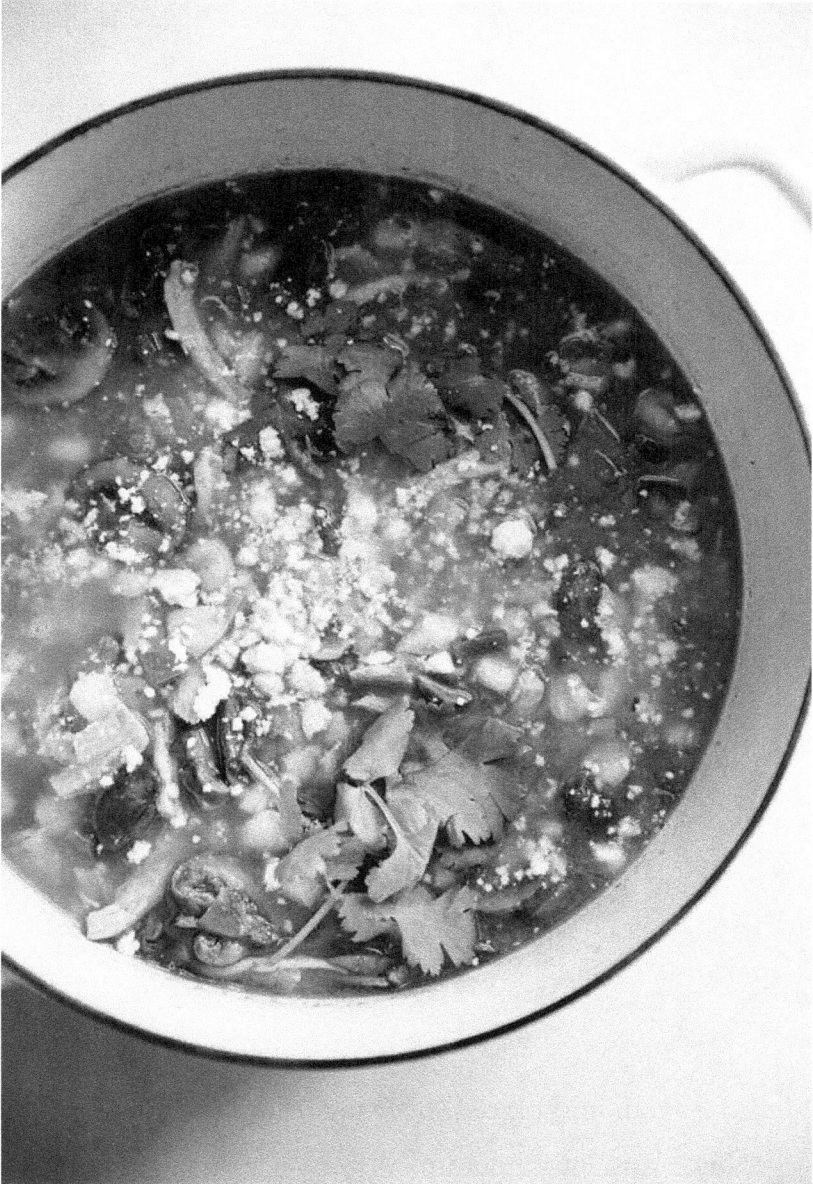

Serving: 2

Prep Time: 10 minutes

Cook Time: Nil

Ingredients:

- 10 ounces chicken livers

- 1-ounce onion, chopped

- 2 ounces sour cream

- 1 tablespoon olive oil

- Sunflower seeds to taste

How To:

1. Take a pan and place it over medium heat.
2. Add oil and let it heat up.
3. Add onions and fry until just browned.

4. Add livers and season with sunflower seeds.

5. Cook until livers are half cooked.

6. Transfer the combination to a stew pot.

7. Add soured cream and cook for 20 minutes.

8. Serve and enjoy!

Nutrition (Per Serving)

Calories: 146

Fat: 9g

Carbohydrates: 2g

Protein: 15g

Chicken Quesadilla

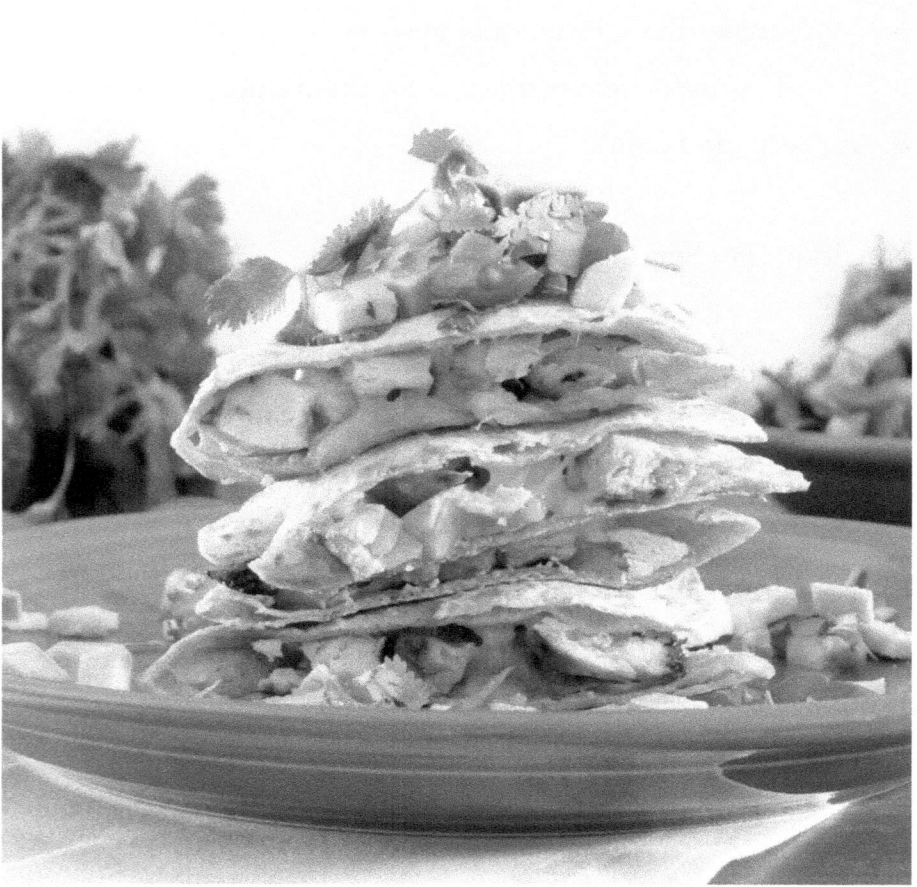

Serving: 2

Prep Time: 10 minutes

Cook Time: 35 minutes

Ingredients:

- ¼ cup ranch dressing

- ½ cup cheddar cheese, shredded

- 20 slices bacon, center-cut

- 2 cups grilled chicken, sliced

How To:

1.   Re-heat your oven to 400 degrees F.

2.   Line baking sheet using parchment paper.

3.   Weave bacon into two rectangles and bake for half-hour .

4.   Lay grilled chicken over bacon square, drizzling ranch dressing on top.

5.   Sprinkle cheddar and top with another bacon square.

6.   Bake for five minutes more.

7.   Slice and serve.

8.   Enjoy!

Nutrition (Per Serving)

Calories: 619

Fat: 35g

Carbohydrates: 2g

Protein: 79g

Mustard Chicken

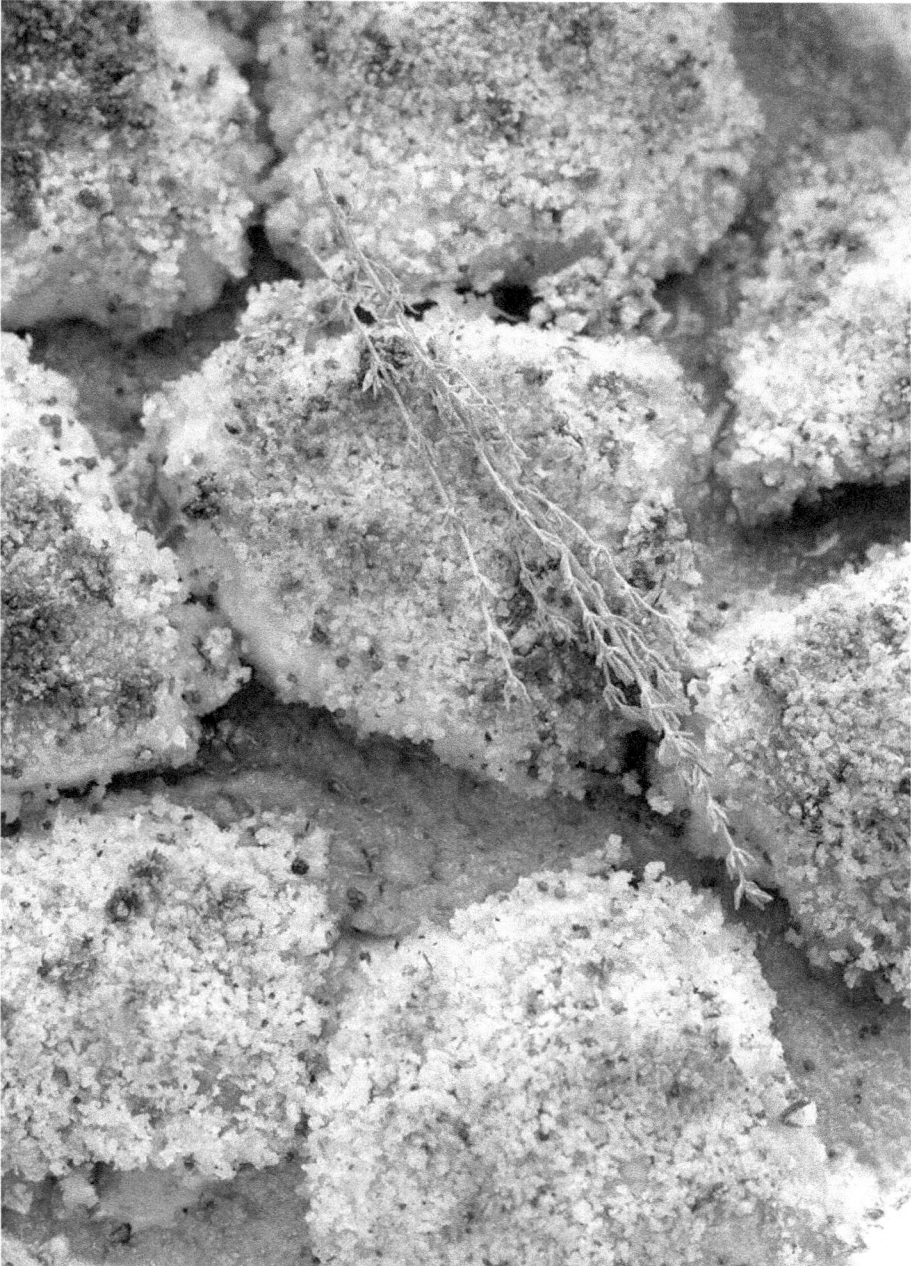

Serving: 2

Prep Time: 10 minutes

Cook Time: 40 minutes

Ingredients:

- 2 chicken breasts

- 1/4 cup chicken broth

- 2 tablespoons mustard

- 1 1/2 tablespoons olive oil

- 1/2 teaspoon paprika

- 1/2 teaspoon chili powder

- 1/2 teaspoon garlic powder

How To:

1.   Take alittle bowl and blend mustard, olive oil, paprika, chicken stock , garlic powder, chicken stock , and chili.

2.   Add pigeon breast and marinate for half-hour .

3.   Take a lined baking sheet and arrange the chicken.

4.   Bake for 35 minutes at 375 degrees F.

5.   Serve and enjoy!

Nutrition (Per Serving)

Calories: 531

Fat: 23g

Carbohydrates: 10g

Protein: 64g

Chicken and Carrot Stew

Serving: 4

Prep Time: 15 minutes

Cook Time: 6 hours

Ingredients:

- 4 boneless chicken breast, cubed

- 3 cups of carrots, peeled and cubed

- 1 cup onion, chopped

- 1 cup tomatoes, chopped

- 1 teaspoon of dried thyme

- 2 cups of chicken broth

- 2 garlic cloves, minced

- Sunflower seeds and pepper as needed

How To:

1. Add all of the listed ingredients to a Slow Cooker.

2. Stir and shut the lid.
3. Cook for six hours.
4. Serve hot and enjoy!

Nutrition (Per Serving)

Calories: 182

Fat: 3g

Carbohydrates: 10g

Protein: 39g

The Delish Turkey Wrap

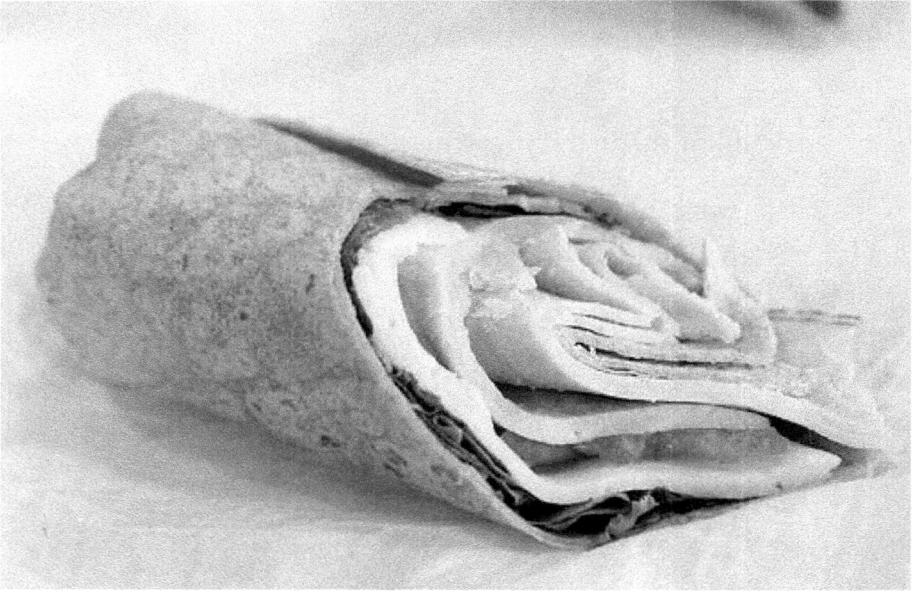

Serving: 6

Prep Time: 10 minutes

Cook Time: 10 minutes

Ingredients:

- 1 ¼ pounds ground turkey, lean

- 4 green onions, minced

- 1 tablespoon olive oil

- 1 garlic clove, minced

- 2 teaspoons chili paste

- 8-ounce water chestnut, diced

- 3 tablespoons hoisin sauce
- 2 tablespoon coconut aminos
- 1 tablespoon rice vinegar

- 12 almond butter lettuce leaves

- 1/8 teaspoon sunflower seeds

How To:

1. Take a pan and place it over medium heat, add turkey and garlic to the pan.

2. Heat for six minutes until cooked.

3. Take a bowl and transfer turkey to the bowl.

4. Add onions and water chestnuts.

5. Stir in duck sauce , coconut aminos, vinegar and chili paste.

6. Toss well and transfer mix to lettuce leaves.

7.   Serve and enjoy!

Nutrition (Per Serving)

Calories: 162

Fat: 4g

Net Carbohydrates: 7g

Protein: 23g

Almond butternut Chicken

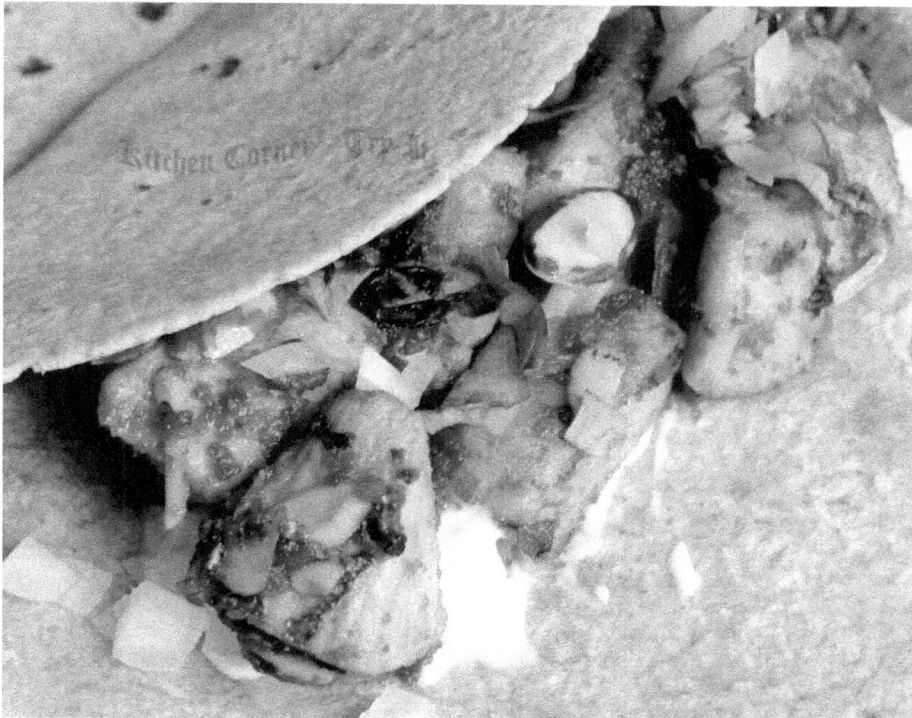

Serving: 4

Prep Time: 15 minutes

Cook Time: 30 minutes

Ingredients:

- ½ pound Nitrate free bacon

- 6 chicken thighs, boneless and skinless

- 2-3 cups almond butternut squash, cubed Extra virgin olive oil Fresh chopped sage

- Sunflower seeds and pepper as needed

How To:

1.   Prepare your oven by preheating it to 425 degrees F.

2.   Take an outsized skillet and place it over medium-high heat, add bacon and fry until crispy.

3.   Take a slice of bacon and place it on the side, crumble the bacon.

4.   Add cubed almond butternut squash within the bacon grease and sauté, season with sunflower seeds and pepper.

5.   Once the squash is tender, remove skillet and transfer to a plate.

6.   Add copra oil to the skillet and add chicken thighs, cook for 10 minutes.

7.   Season with sunflower seeds and pepper.

8.   Remove skillet from stove and transfer to oven.

9.   Bake for 12-15 minutes, top with the crumbled bacon and sage.

10. Enjoy!

Nutrition (Per Serving)

Calories: 323

Fat: 19g

Carbohydrates: 8g

Protein: 12g

Zucchini Zoodles with Chicken and Basil

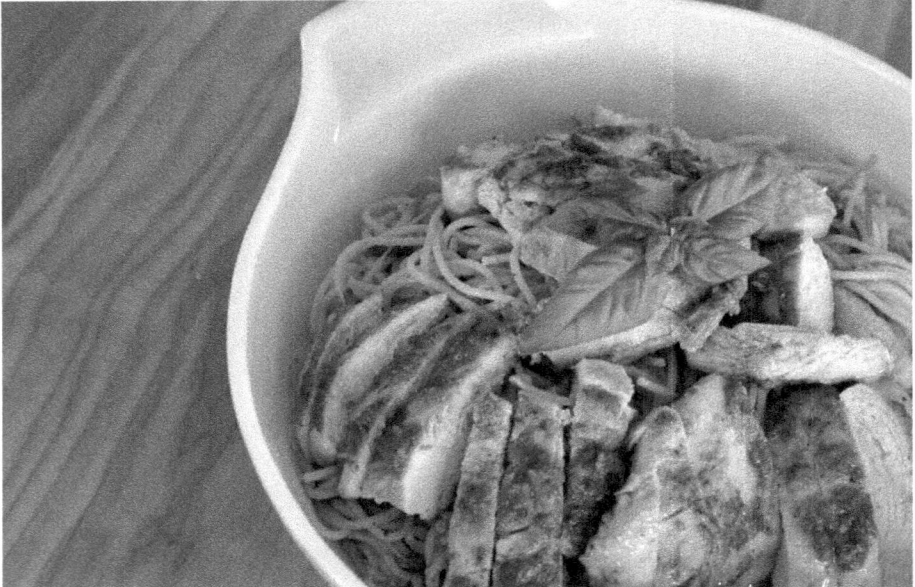

Serving: 3

Prep Time: 10 minutes

Cook Time: 10 minutes

Ingredients:

2 chicken fillets, cubed

2 tablespoons ghee

1-pound tomatoes, diced

½ cup basil, chopped

¼ cup almond milk

1 garlic clove, peeled, minced

1 zucchini, shredded

How To:

1.   Sauté cubed chicken in ghee until not pink.

2.   Add tomatoes and season with sunflower seeds.

3.   Simmer and reduce liquid.

4.   Prepare your zucchini Zoodles by shredding zucchini during a kitchen appliance .

5.   Add basil, garlic, coconut almond milk to the chicken and cook for a couple of minutes.

6.   Add half the zucchini Zoodles to a bowl and top with creamy tomato basil chicken.

7.   Enjoy!

Nutrition (Per Serving)

Calories: 540

Fat: 27g

Carbohydrates: 13g

Protein: 59g

Duck with Cucumber and Carrots

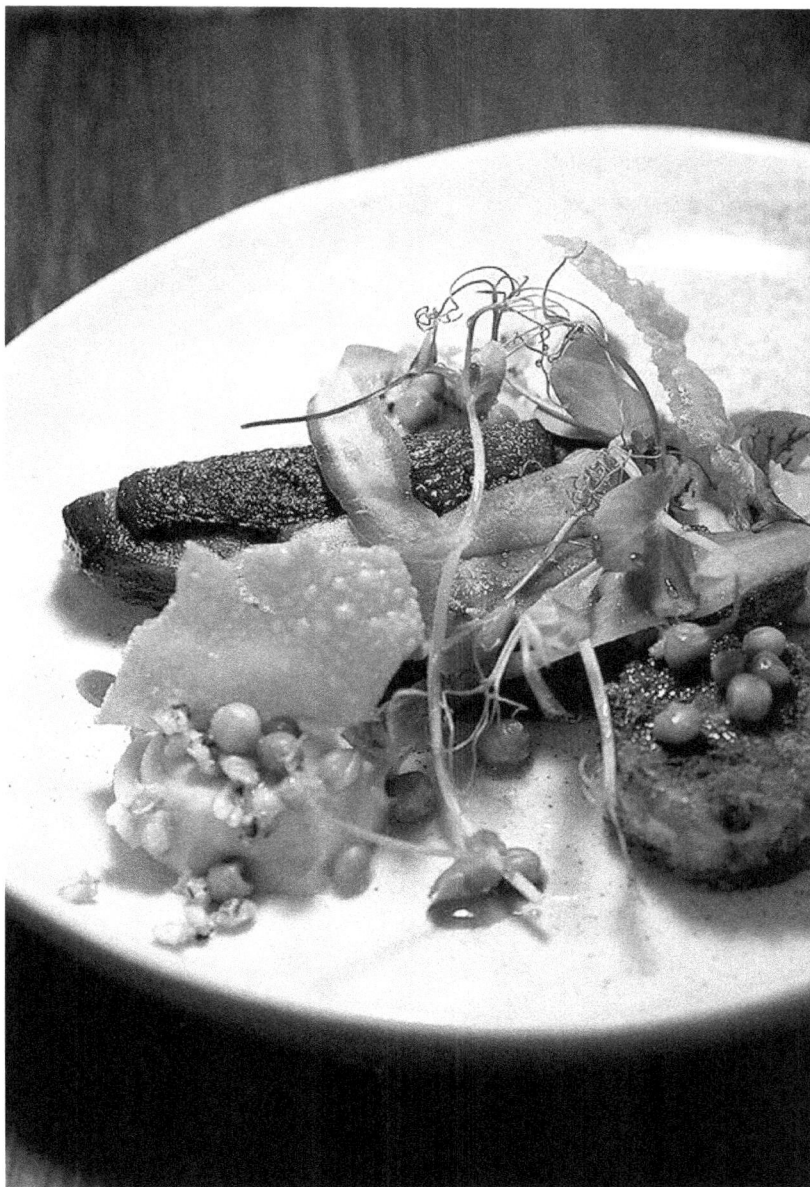

Serving: 8

Prep Time: 10 minutes

Cook Time: 40 minutes

Ingredients:

- 1 duck, cut up into medium pieces

- 1 chopped cucumber, chopped

- 1 tablespoon low sodium vegetable stock

- 2 carrots, chopped

- 2 cups of water

- Black pepper as needed

- 1-inch ginger piece, grated

How To:

1.   Add duck pieces to your Instant Pot.

2.   Add cucumber, stock, carrots, water, ginger, pepper and stir.

3.   Lock up the lid and cook on low for 40 minutes.

4.   Release the pressure naturally.

5.   Serve and enjoy!

Nutrition (Per Serving)

Calories: 206

Fats: 7g

Carbs: 28g

Protein: 16g

Parmesan Baked Chicken

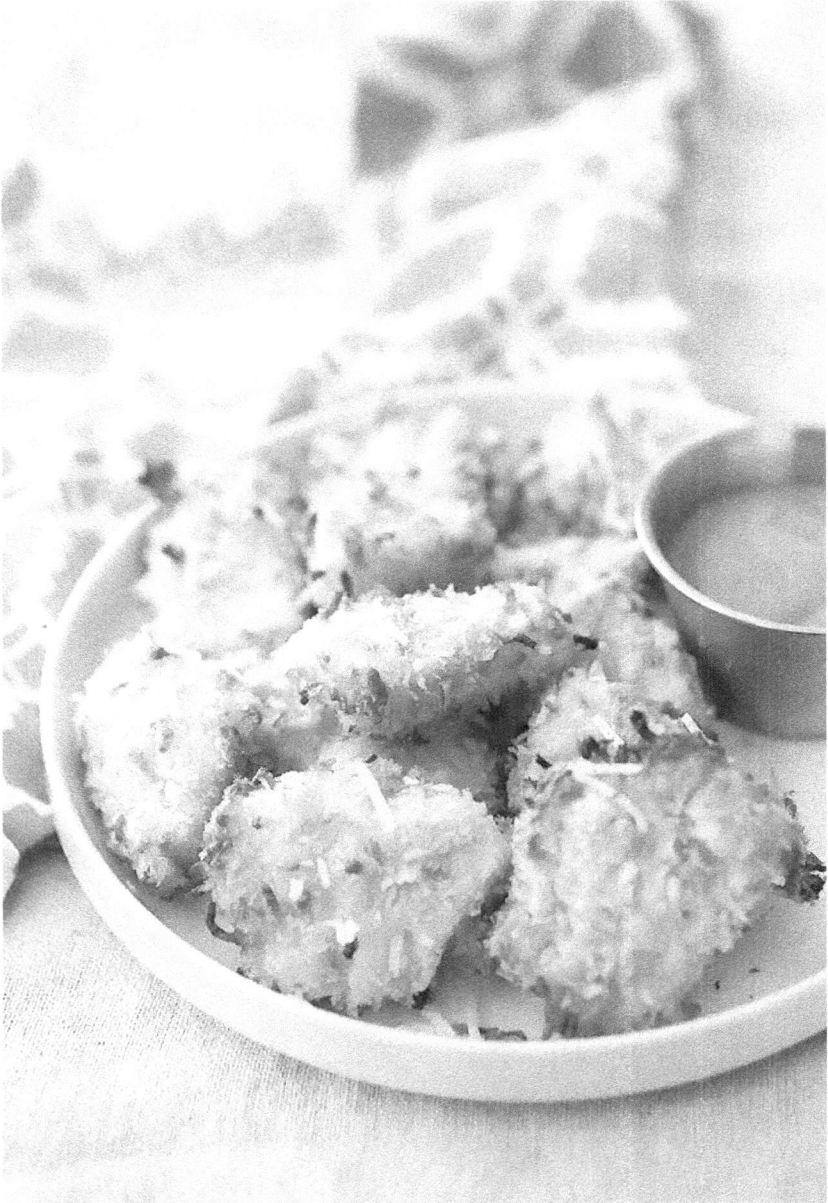

Serving: 2

Prep Time: 5 minutes

Cook Time: 20 minutes

Ingredients:

- 2 tablespoons ghee

- 2 boneless chicken breasts, skinless

- Pink sunflower seeds

- Freshly ground black pepper

- ½ cup mayonnaise, low fat

- ¼ cup parmesan cheese, grated

- 1 tablespoon dried Italian seasoning, low fat, low sodium ¼ cup crushed pork rinds

How To:

1. Preheat your oven to 425 degrees F.

2. Take an outsized baking dish and coat with ghee.

3. Pat chicken breasts dry and wrap with a towel.

4. Season with sunflower seeds and pepper.

5. Place in baking dish.

6. Take alittle bowl and add mayonnaise, parmesan cheese, Italian seasoning.

7. Slather mayo mix evenly over pigeon breast .

8. Sprinkle crushed pork rinds on top.

9. Bake for 20 minutes until topping is browned.

10. Serve and enjoy!

Nutrition (Per Serving)

Calories: 850

Fat: 67g

Carbohydrates: 2g

Protein: 60g

Buffalo Chicken Lettuce Wraps

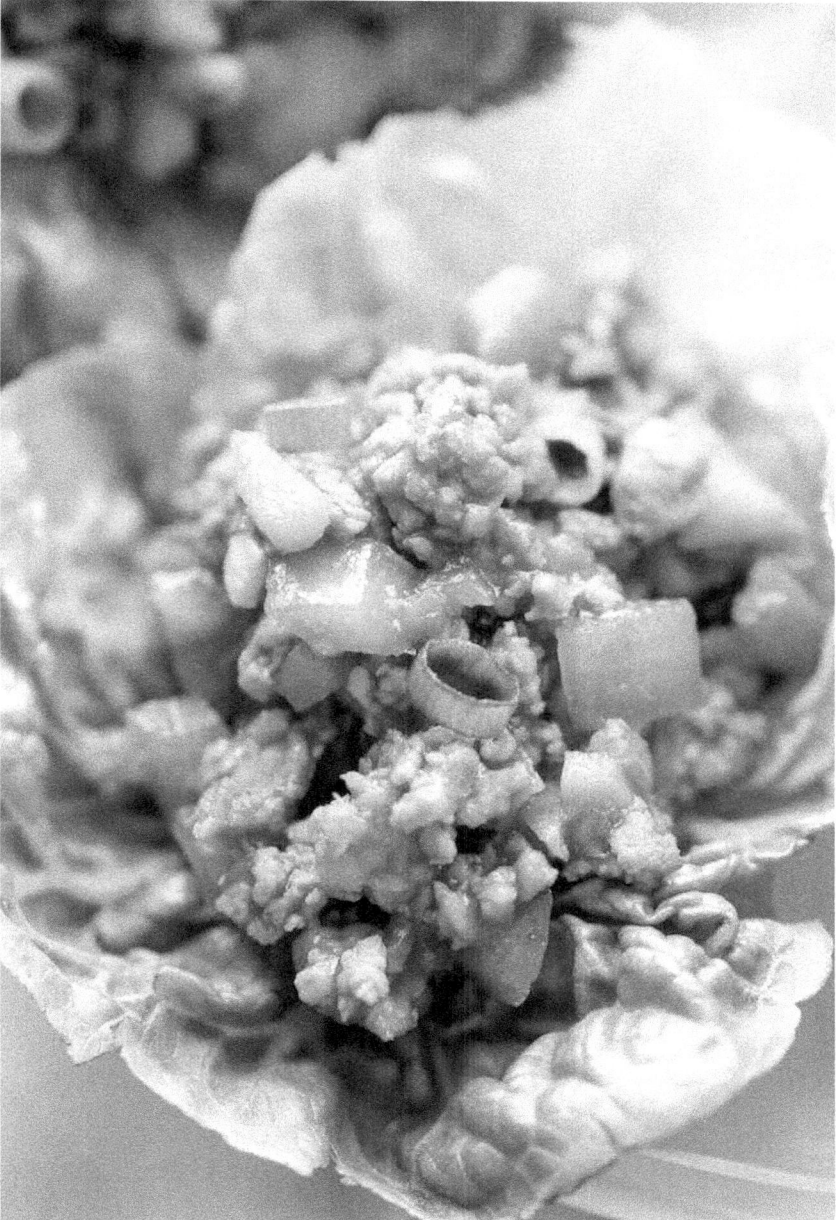

Serving: 2

Prep Time: 35 minutes

Cook Time: 10 minutes

Ingredients:

- 3 chicken breasts, boneless and cubed

- 20 slices of almond butter lettuce leaves

- ¾ cup cherry tomatoes halved

- 1 avocado, chopped

- ¼ cup green onions, diced

- ½ cup ranch dressing

- ¾ cup hot sauce

How To:

1. Take a bowl and add chicken cubes and sauce , mix.

2.   Place within the fridge and let it marinate for half-hour .

3.   Preheat your oven to 400 degrees F.

4.   Place coated chicken on a cookie pan and bake for 9 minutes.

5.   Assemble lettuce serving cups with equal amounts of lettuce, green onions, tomatoes, ranch dressing, and cubed chicken.

6.   Serve and enjoy!

Nutrition (Per Serving)

Calories: 106

Fat: 6g

Net Carbohydrates: 2g

Protein: 5g

Crazy Japanese Potato and Beef Croquettes

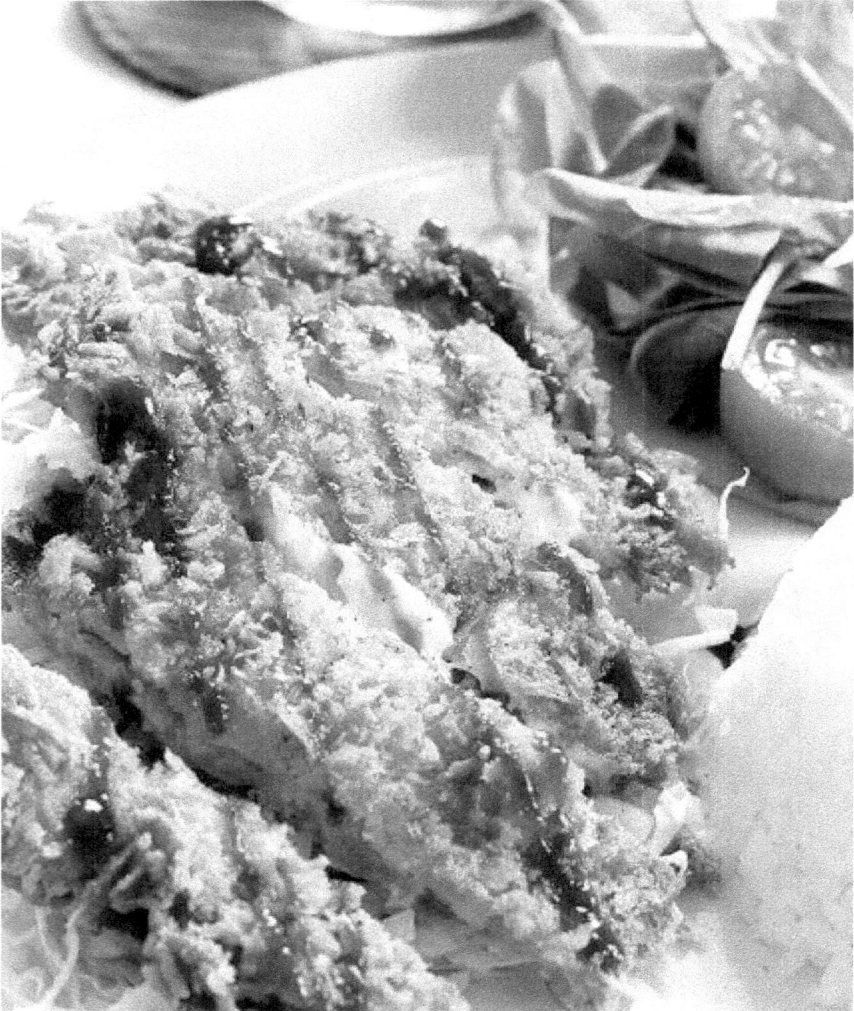

Serving: 10

Prep Time: 10 minute

Cook Time: 20 minutes

Ingredients:

- 3 medium russet potatoes, peeled and chopped

- 1 tablespoon almond butter

- 1 tablespoon vegetable oil

- 3 onions, diced

- ¾ pound ground beef

- 4 teaspoons light coconut aminos

- All-purpose flour for coating

- 2 eggs, beaten

- Panko bread crumbs for coating

- ½ cup oil, frying

How To:

1.   Take a saucepan and place it over medium-high heat; add potatoes and sunflower seeds water, boil for 16 minutes.

2.   Remove water and put potatoes in another bowl, add almond butter and mash the potatoes.

3.   Take a frypan and place it over medium heat, add 1 tablespoon oil and let it heat up.

4.   Add onions and fry until tender.

5.   Add coconut aminos to beef to onions.

6.   Keep frying until beef is browned.

7.   Mix the meat with the potatoes evenly.

8.   Take another frypan and place it over medium heat; add half a cup of oil.

9.   Form croquettes using the potato mixture and coat them with flour, then eggs and eventually breadcrumbs.

10.   Fry patties until golden on all sides.

11.   Enjoy!

Nutrition (Per Serving)

Calories: 239

Fat: 4g

Carbohydrates: 20g

Protein: 10g

Spicy Chili Crackers

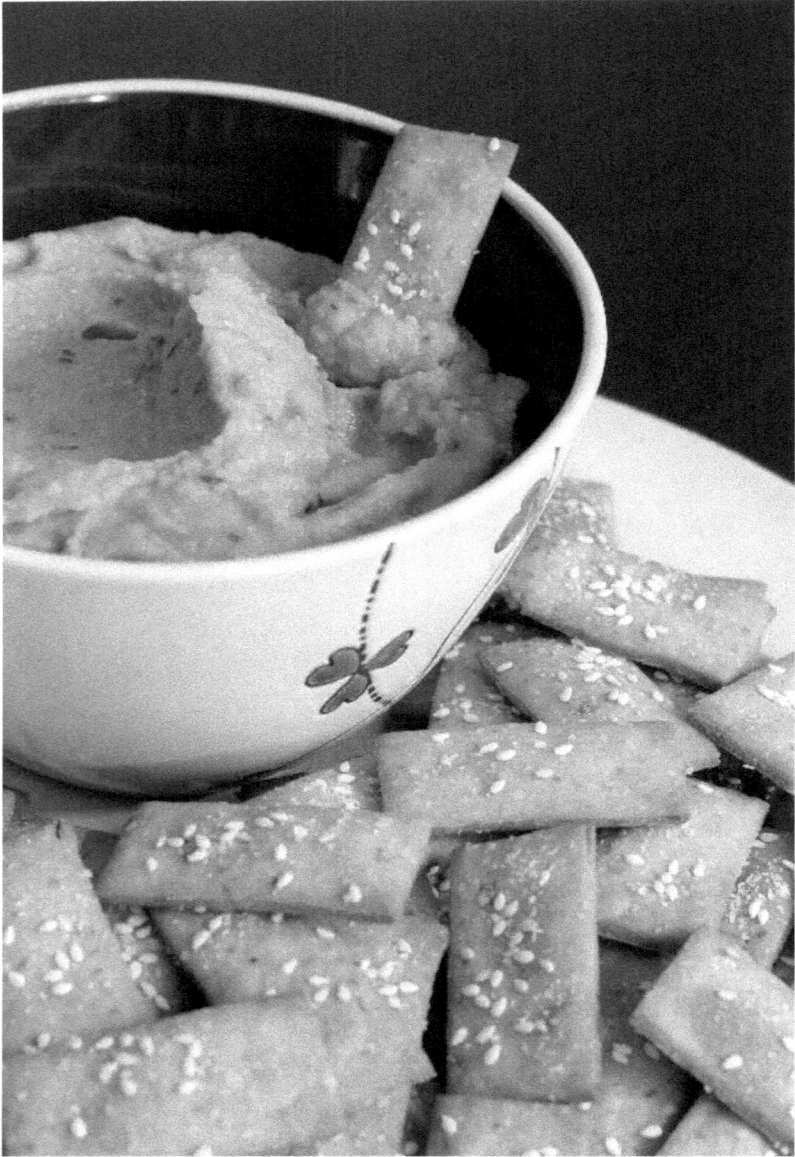

Serving: 30 crackers

Prep Time: 15 minutes

Cooking Time: 60 minutes

Ingredients:

- ¾ cup almond flour

- ¼ cup coconut four

- ¼ cup coconut flour

- ½ teaspoon paprika

- ½ teaspoon cumin

- 1 ½ teaspoons chili pepper spice

- 1 teaspoon onion powder

- ½ teaspoon sunflower seeds

- 1 whole egg

- ¼ cup unsalted almond butter

How To:

1. Preheat your oven to 350 degrees F.

2. Line a baking sheet with parchment paper and keep it on the side.

3. Add ingredients to your kitchen appliance and pulse until you've got a pleasant dough.

4. Divide dough into two equal parts.

5. Place one ball on a sheet of parchment paper and canopy with another sheet; roll it out.

6. dig crackers and repeat with the opposite ball.

7. Transfer the prepped dough to a baking tray and bake for 8-10 minutes.

8. Remove from oven and serve.

9. Enjoy!

Nutrition (Per Serving)

Total Carbs: 2.8g

Fiber: 1g

Protein: 1.6g

Fat: 4.1g

Golden Eggplant Fries

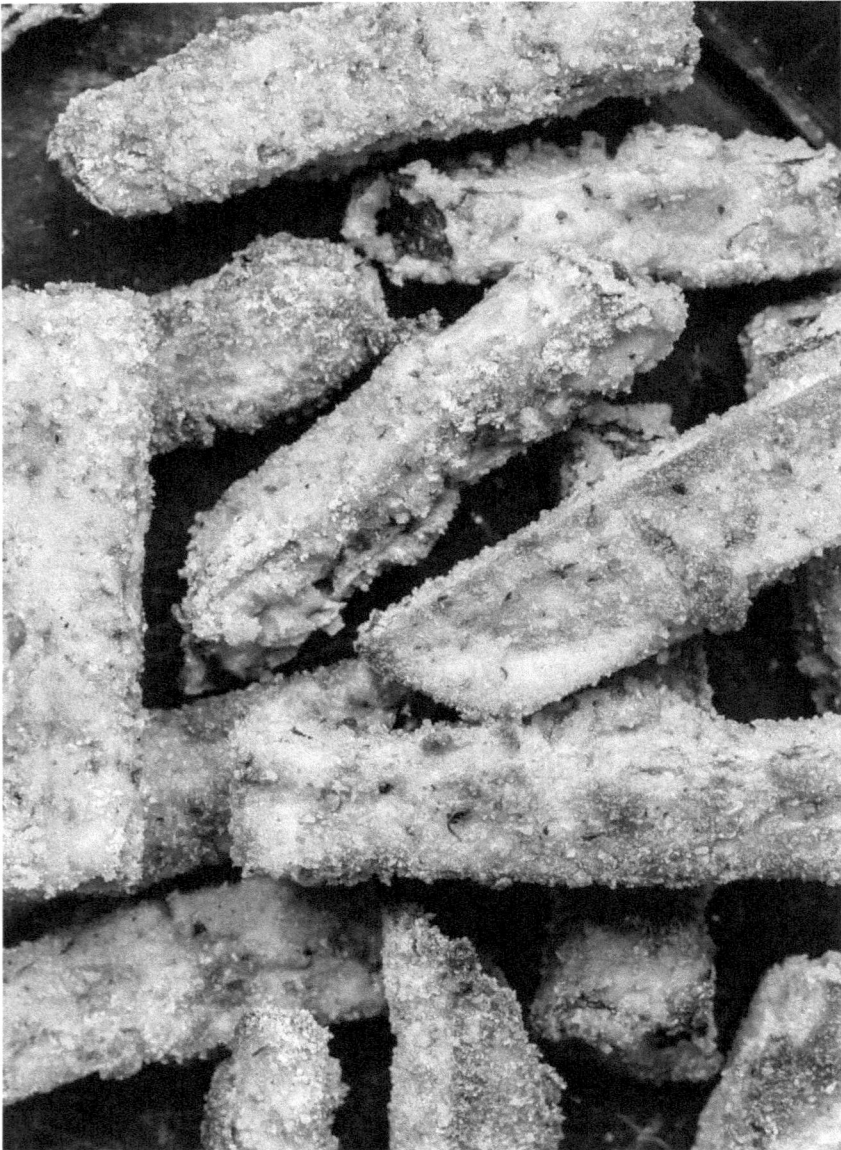

Serving: 8

Prep Time: 10 minutes

Cook Time: 15 minutes

Ingredients:

- 2 eggs

- 2 cups almond flour

- 2 tablespoons coconut oil, spray

- 2 eggplant, peeled and cut thinly Sunflower seeds and pepper

How To:

1.   Preheat your oven to 400 degrees F.

2.   Take a bowl and blend with sunflower seeds and black pepper.

3.   Take another bowl and beat eggs until frothy.

4.   Dip the eggplant pieces into the eggs.

5.   Then coat them with the flour mixture.

6.   Add another layer of flour and egg.

7.   Then, take a baking sheet and grease with copra oil on top.

8.   Bake for about quarter-hour .

9.   Serve and enjoy!

Nutrition (Per Serving)

Calories: 212

Fat: 15.8g

Carbohydrates: 12.1g

Protein: 8.6g

Traditional Black Bean Chili

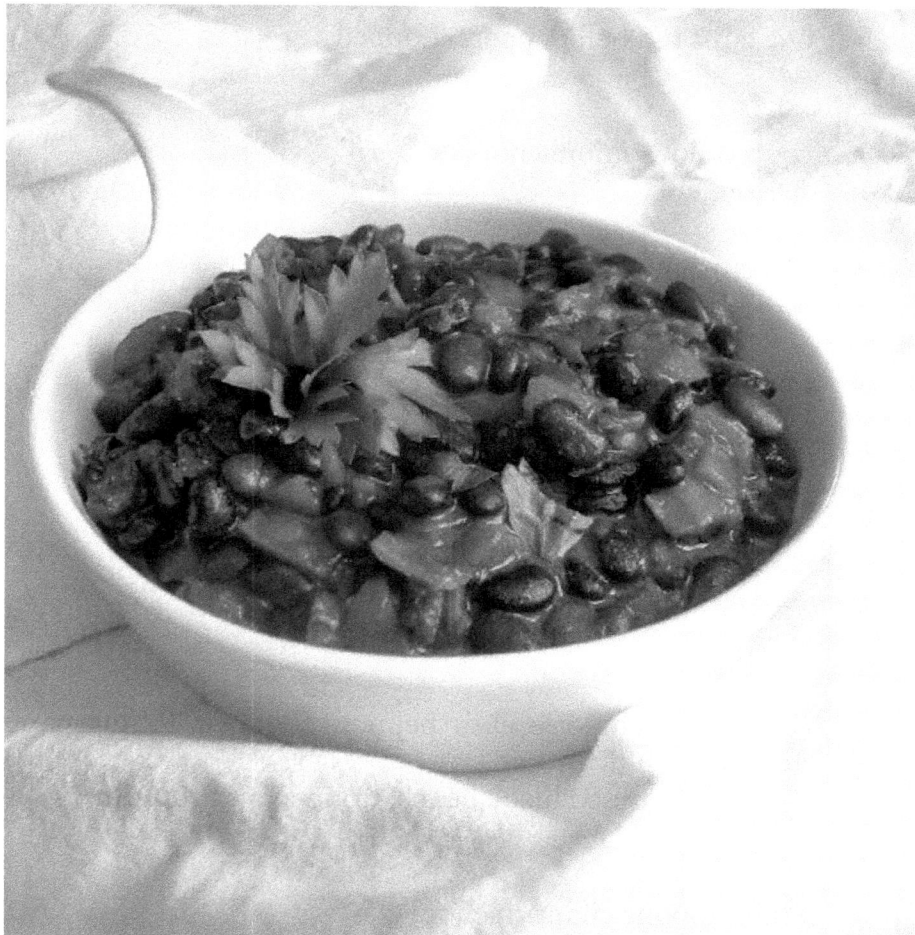

Serving: 4

Prep Time: 10 minutes

Cooking Time: 4 hours

Ingredients:

- 1 ½ cups red bell pepper, chopped

- 1 cup yellow onion, chopped

- 1 ½ cups mushrooms, sliced

- 1 tablespoon olive oil

- 1 tablespoon chili powder

- 2 garlic cloves, minced

- 1 teaspoon chipotle chili pepper, chopped ½ teaspoon cumin, ground
- 16 ounces canned black beans, drained and rinsed

- 2 tablespoons cilantro, chopped

- 1 cup tomatoes, chopped

How To:

1.   Add red bell peppers, onion, dill, mushrooms, flavor, garlic, chili pepper, cumin, black beans, tomatoes to your Slow Cooker.

2.   Stir well.

3.   Place lid and cook on HIGH for 4 hours.

4.   Sprinkle cilantro on top.

5.   Serve and enjoy!

Nutrition (Per Serving)

Calories: 211

Fat: 3g

Carbohydrates: 22g

Protein: 5g

Very Wild Mushroom Pilaf

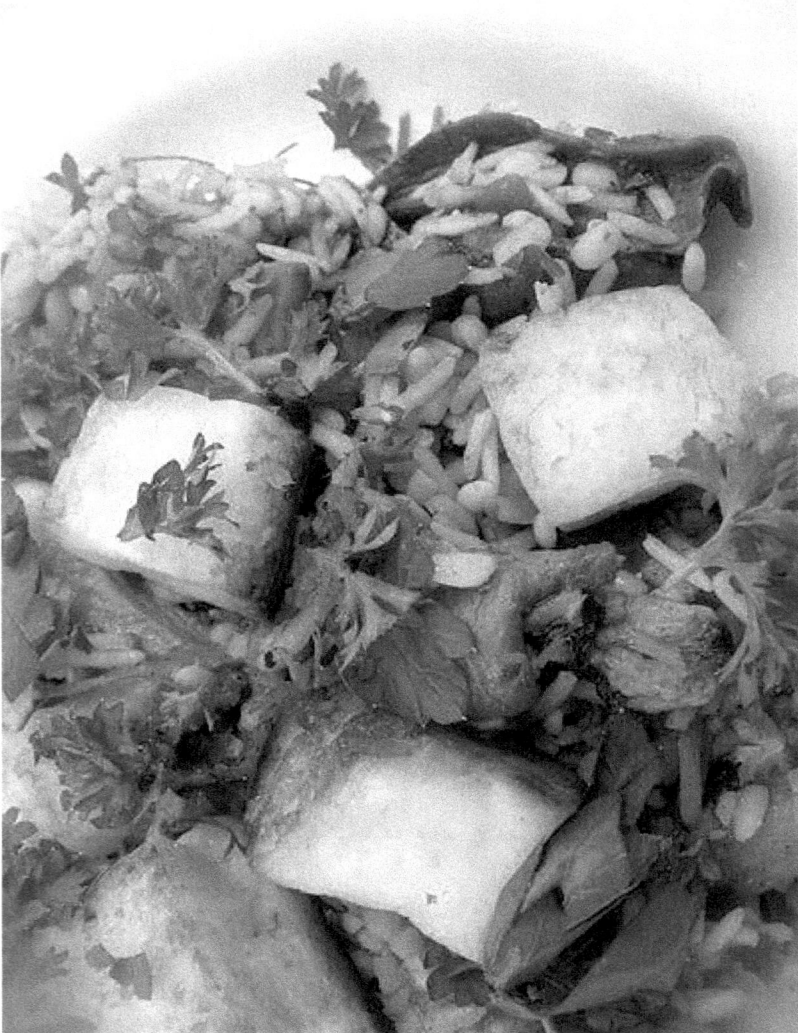

Serving: 4

Prep Time: 10 minutes

Cooking Time: 3 hours

Ingredients:

- 1 cup wild rice

- 2 garlic cloves, minced

- 6 green onions, chopped

- 2 tablespoons olive oil

- ½ pound baby Bella mushrooms

- 2 cups water

How To:

1.   Add rice, garlic, onion, oil, mushrooms and water to your Slow Cooker.

2.   Stir well until mixed.

3.   Place lid and cook on LOW for 3 hours.

4.   Stir pilaf and divide between serving platters.

5.   Enjoy!

Nutrition (Per Serving)

Calories: 210

Fat: 7g

Carbohydrates: 16g

Protein: 4g

Green Palak Paneer

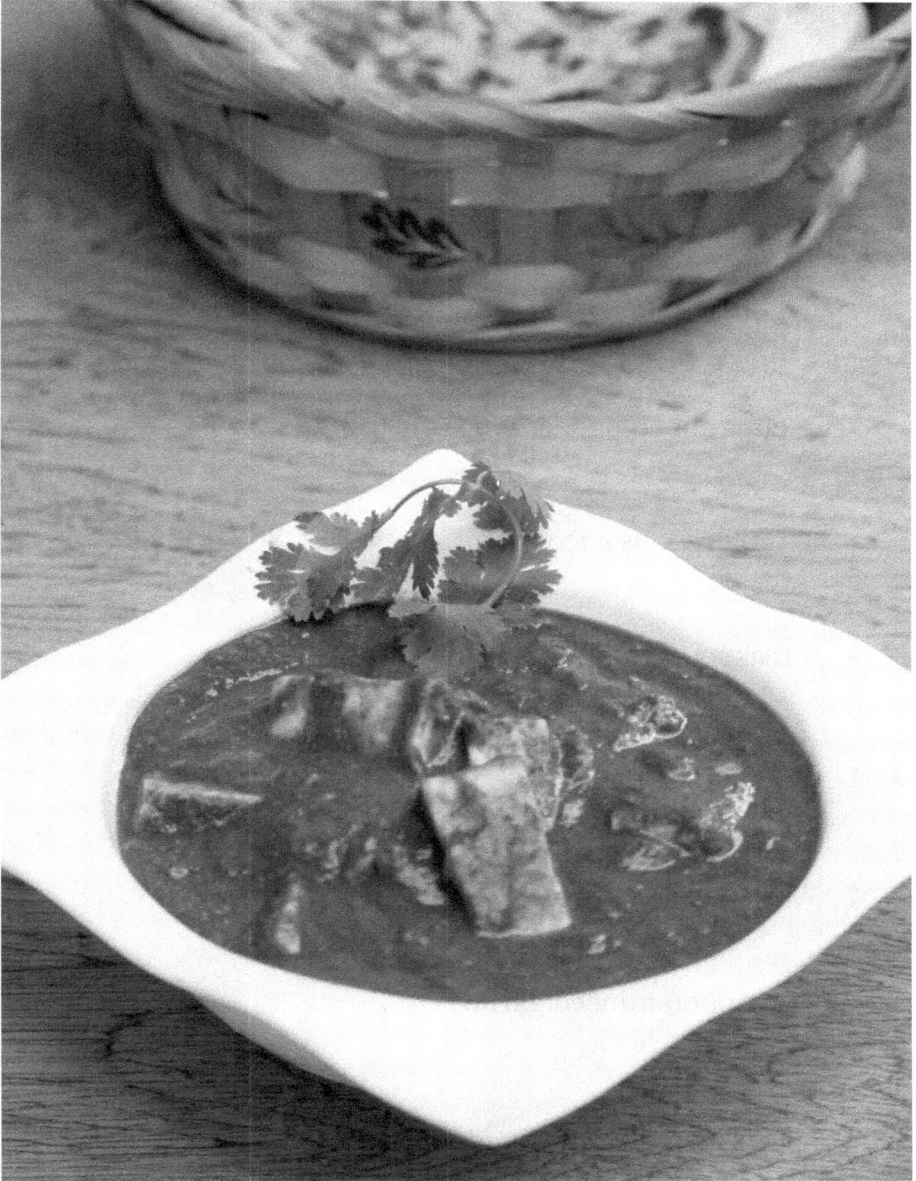

Serving: 4

Prep Time: 5 minutes

Cook Time: 10 minutes

Ingredients:

- 1-pound spinach

- 2 cups cubed paneer (vegan)

- 2 tablespoons coconut oil

- 1 teaspoon cumin

- 1 chopped up onion

- 1-2 teaspoons hot green chili minced up

- 1 teaspoon minced garlic

- 15 cashews

- 4 tablespoons almond milk

- 1 teaspoon Garam masala

- Flavored vinegar as needed

How To:

1.   Add cashews and milk to a blender and blend well.

2.   Set your pot to Sauté mode and add coconut oil; allow the oil to heat up.

3.   Add cumin seeds, garlic, green chilies, ginger and sauté for 1 minute.

4.   Add onion and sauté for two minutes.

5.   Add chopped spinach, flavored vinegar and a cup of water.

6.   Lock up the lid and cook on high for 10 minutes.

7.   Quick-release the pressure.

8.   Add ½ cup of water and blend to a paste.

9.   Add cashew paste, paneer and Garam Masala and stir thoroughly.

10.   Serve over hot rice!

Nutrition (Per Serving)

Calories: 367

Fat: 26g

Carbohydrates: 21g

Protein: 16g

Sporty Baby Carrots

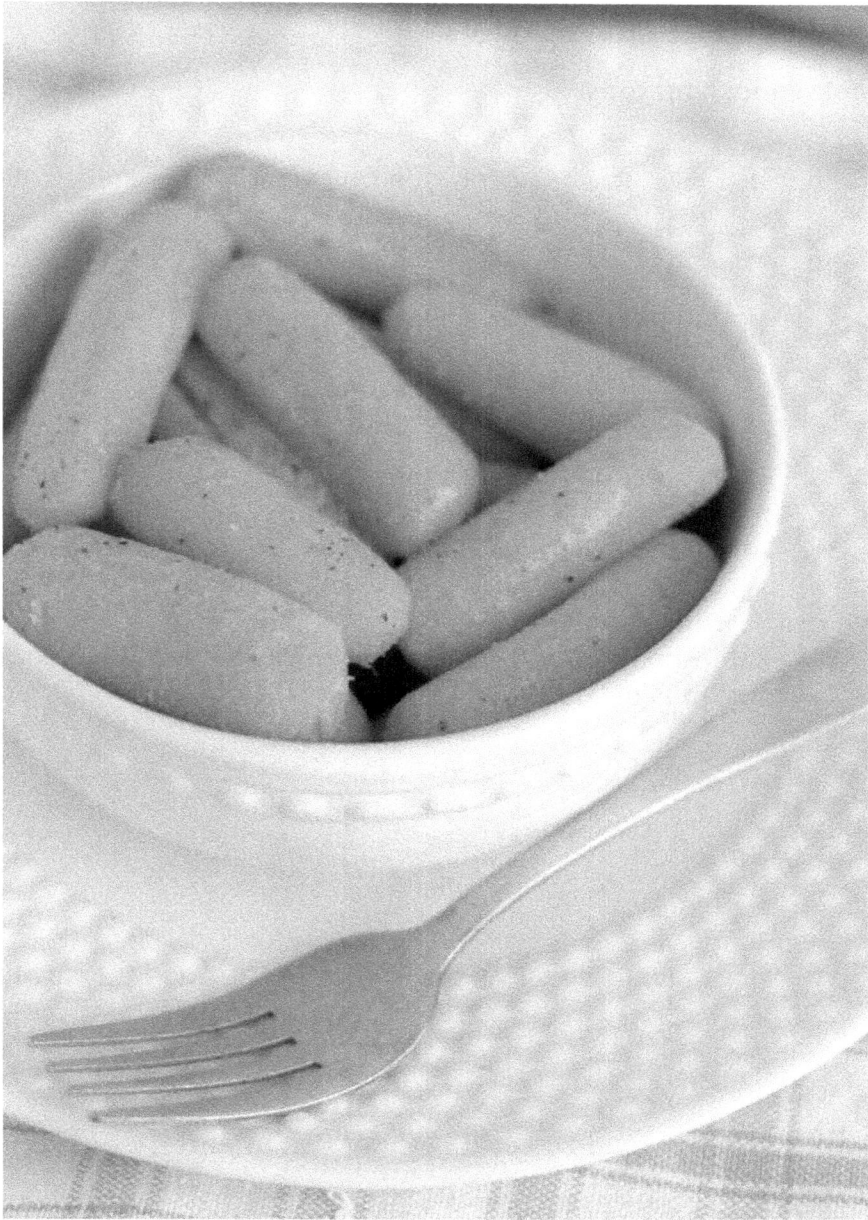

Serving: 4

Prep Time: 5 minutes

Cook Time: 5 minutes

Ingredients:

- 1-pound baby carrots

- 1 cup water

- 1 tablespoon clarified ghee

- 1 tablespoon chopped up fresh mint leaves Sea flavored vinegar as needed

How To:

1.   Place a steamer rack on top of your pot and add the carrots.

2.   Add water .

3.   Lock the lid and cook at high for two minutes.

4.   Do a fast release.

5.   Pass the carrots through a strainer and drain them.

6.   Wipe the insert clean.

7.   Return the insert to the pot and set the pot to Sauté mode.

8.   Add drawn butter and permit it to melt.

9.   Add mint and sauté for 30 seconds.

10.   Add carrots to the insert and sauté well.

11.   Remove them and sprinkle with little bit of flavored vinegar on top.

12.   Enjoy!

Nutrition (Per Serving)

Calories: 131

Fat: 10g

Carbohydrates: 11g

Protein: 1g

Saucy Garlic Greens

Serving: 4

Prep Time: 5 minutes

Cook Time: 20 minutes

Ingredients:

- 1 bunch of leafy greens Sauce

- ½ cup cashews soaked in water for 10 minutes ¼ cup water

- 1 tablespoon lemon juice

- 1 teaspoon coconut aminos

- 1 clove peeled whole clove

- 1/8 teaspoon of flavored vinegar

How To:

1.   Make the sauce by draining and discarding the soaking water from your cashews and add the cashews to a blender.

2.   Add water , juice , flavored vinegar, coconut aminos, garlic.

3.   Blitz until you've got a smooth cream and transfer to bowl.

4.   Add ½ cup of water to the pot.

5.   Place the steamer basket to the pot and add the greens within the basket.

6.   Lock the lid and steam for 1 minute.

7.   Quick-release the pressure.

8.   Transfer the steamed greens to strainer and extract excess water.

9.   Place the greens into a bowl .

10.   Add lemon aioli and toss.

11.   Enjoy!

Nutrition (Per Serving)

Calories: 77

Fat: 5g

Carbohydrates: 0g

Protein: 2g

Garden Salad

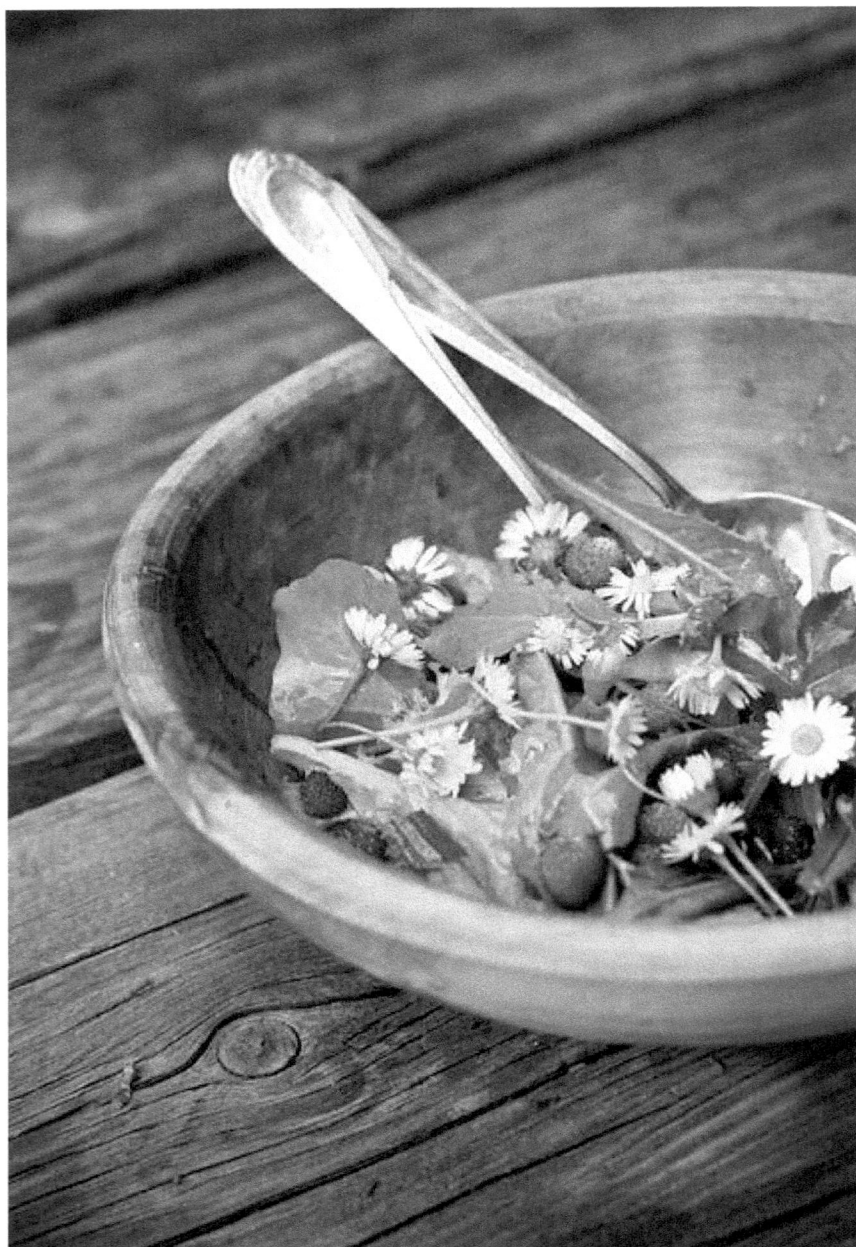

Serving: 6

Prep Time: 5 minutes

Cook Time: 20 minutes

Ingredients:

- 1 pound raw peanuts in shell

- 1 bay leaf

- 2 medium-sized chopped up tomatoes

- ½ cup diced up green pepper

- ½ cup diced up sweet onion

- ¼ cup finely diced hot pepper

- ¼ cup diced up celery

- 2 tablespoons olive oil

- ¾ teaspoon flavored vinegar

- ¼ teaspoon freshly ground black pepper

How To:

1. Boil your peanuts for 1 minute and rinse them.
2. The skin are going to be soft, so discard the skin.
3. Add 2 cups of water to the moment Pot.
4. Add herb and peanuts.
5. Lock the lid and cook on high for 20 minutes.
6. Drain the water.
7. Take an outsized bowl and add the peanuts, diced up vegetables.
8. Whisk in vegetable oil , juice , pepper in another bowl.
9. Pour the mixture over the salad and blend .
10. Enjoy!

Nutrition (Per Serving)

Calories: 140

Fat: 4g

Carbohydrates: 24g

Protein: 5g

Spicy Cabbage Dish

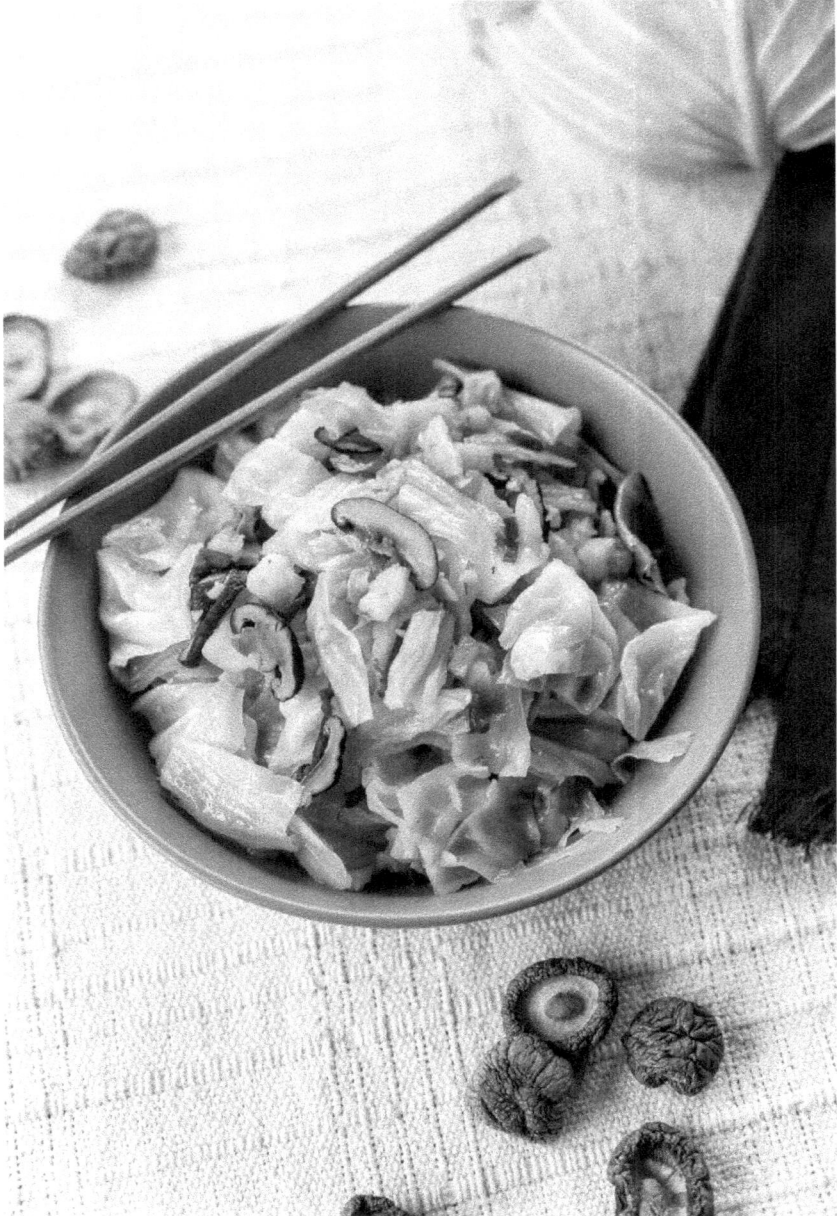

Serving: 4

Prep Time: 10 minutes

Cooking Time: 4 hours

Ingredients:

- 2 yellow onions, chopped

- 10 cups red cabbage, shredded

- 1 cup plums, pitted and chopped

- 1 teaspoon cinnamon powder

- 1 garlic clove, minced

- 1 teaspoon cumin seeds

- ¼ teaspoon cloves, ground

- 2 tablespoons red wine vinegar

- 1 teaspoon coriander seeds

- ½ cup water

How To:

1.	Add cabbage, onion, plums, garlic, cumin, cinnamon, cloves, vinegar, coriander and water to your Slow Cooker.

2.	Stir well.

3.	Place lid and cook on LOW for 4 hours.

4.	Divide between serving platters.

5.	Enjoy!

Nutrition (Per Serving)

Calories: 197

Fat: 1g

Carbohydrates: 14g

Protein: 3g

Extreme Balsamic Chicken

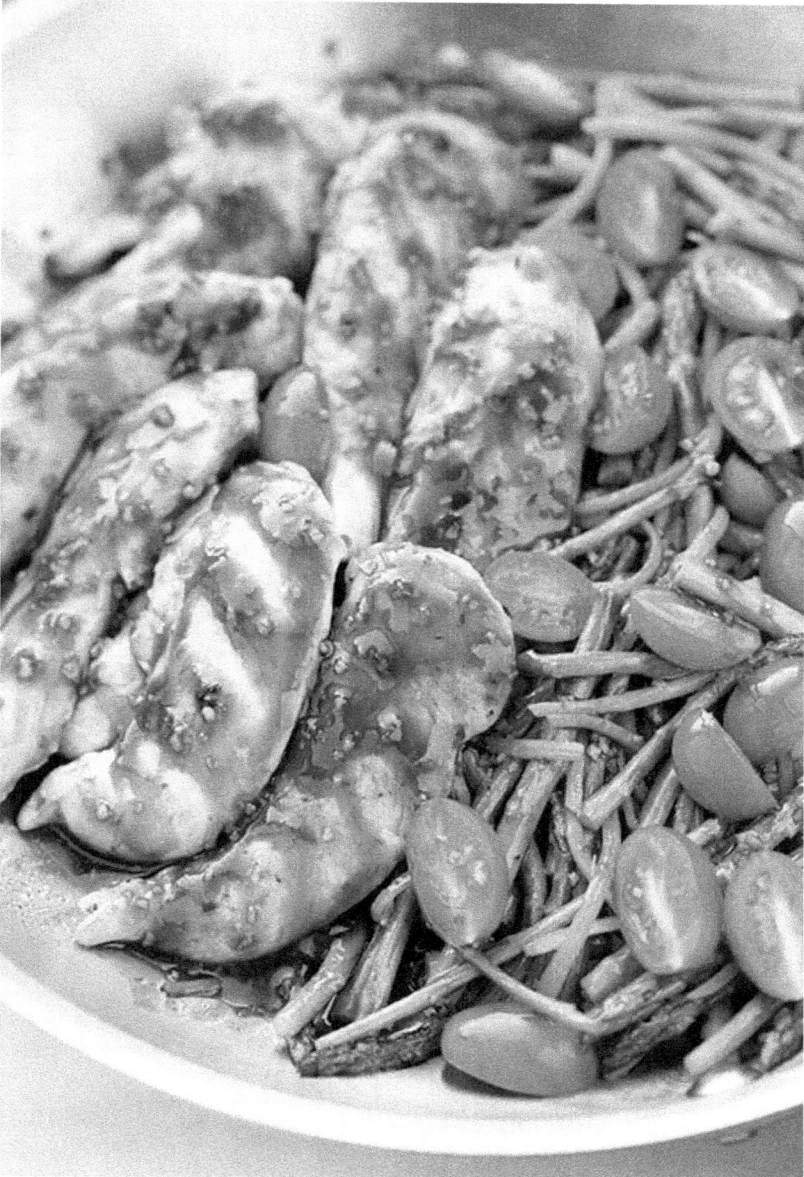

Serving: 4

Prep Time: 10 minutes

Cook Time: 35 minutes

Ingredients:

- 3 boneless chicken breasts, skinless

- Sunflower seeds to taste

- ¼ cup almond flour

- 2/3 cups low-fat chicken broth

- 1 ½ teaspoons arrowroot

- ½ cup low sugar raspberry preserve

- 1 ½ tablespoons balsamic vinegar

How To:

1.   Cut pigeon breast into bite-sized pieces and season them with seeds.

2.   Dredge the chicken pieces in flour and shake off any excess.

3.   Take a non-stick skillet and place it over medium heat.

4.   Add chicken to the skillet and cook for quarter-hour , ensuring to show them half-way through.

5.   Remove chicken and transfer to platter.

6.   Add arrowroot, broth, raspberry preserve to the skillet and stir.

7.   Stir in balsamic vinegar and reduce heat to low, stir-cook for a couple of minutes.

8.   Transfer the chicken back to the sauce and cook for quarter-hour more.

9.   Serve and enjoy!

Nutrition (Per Serving)

Calories: 546

Fat: 35g

Carbohydrates: 11g

Protein: 44g

www.ingramcontent.com/pod-product-compliance
Lightning Source LLC
Chambersburg PA
CBHW070722030426

42336CB00013B/1887